Strong Arms & Upper Body

JOE WUEBBEN

JIM STOPPANI, PhD

Library of Congress Cataloging-in-Publication Data

Wuebben, Joe.
  Stronger arms & upper body / Joe Wuebben, Jim Stoppani.
    p. cm.
  ISBN-13: 978-0-7360-7401-8 (soft cover)
  ISBN-10: 0-7360-7401-5 (soft cover)
  1. Exercise. 2. Arm exercises. 3. Bodybuilding. I. Stoppani, James,
1968- II. Title.
  GV508.W84 2009
  613.7--dc22

                              2008024798

  ISBN-10: 0-7360-7401-5
  ISBN-13: 978-0-7360-7401-8

Acquisitions Editor: Justin Klug; **Developmental Editor:** Heather Healy; **Assistant Editor:** Carla Zych; **Copyeditor:** Jan Feeney; **Proofreader:** Coree Clark; **Permission Manager:** Martha Gullo; **Graphic Designer:** Robert Reuther; **Graphic Artist:** Kim McFarland; **Cover Designer:** Keith Blomberg; **Photographer (cover and interior):** Neil Bernstein; **Photo Office Assistant:** Jason Allen; **Art Manager:** Kelly Hendren; **Associate Art Manager:** Alan L. Wilborn; **Illustrator:** Jason McAlexander; **Printer:** United Graphics

We thank International Sportscience Institute in West Los Angeles, California, and Powerhouse Gym in Chatsworth, California, for assistance in providing the locations for the photo shoot for this book. We thank the photo shoot models: Matus Valent, Christian Ramirez, and Nola Trimble.

Human Kinetics books are available at special discounts for bulk purchase. Special editions or book excerpts can also be created to specification. For details, contact the Special Sales Manager at Human Kinetics.

Printed in the United States of America   10 9 8 7 6 5 4 3 2 1

Human Kinetics
Web site: www.HumanKinetics.com

United States: Human Kinetics
P.O. Box 5076
Champaign, IL 61825-5076
800-747-4457
e-mail: humank@hkusa.com

Canada: Human Kinetics
475 Devonshire Road Unit 100
Windsor, ON N8Y 2L5
800-465-7301 (in Canada only)
e-mail: info@hkcanada.com

Europe: Human Kinetics
107 Bradford Road
Stanningley
Leeds LS28 6AT, United Kingdom
+44 (0) 113 255 5665
e-mail: hk@hkeurope.com

Australia: Human Kinetics
57A Price Avenue
Lower Mitcham, South Australia 5062
08 8372 0999
e-mail: info@hkaustralia.com

New Zealand: Human Kinetics
Division of Sports Distributors NZ Ltd.
P.O. Box 300 226 Albany
North Shore City
Auckland
0064 9 448 1207
e-mail: info@humankinetics.co.nz

Contents

Introduction

There's a reason that new cars, televisions, and cell phones come with owner's manuals. Because of the complexity of the products, managing and maintaining a machine are anything but self-explanatory. The human body is similar in this regard, except that it's far more complex than even the most cutting-edge piece of technology—far too intricate to try to maintain, and more specifically *improve,* through weight training without some sort of reference guide. Thus, you can think of this book as an owner's manual for training your arms and upper body.

A good owner's manual is easy to follow and is written with the utmost clarity and efficiency. One thing we strived for in this book was to eliminate all trivial information; in other words, everything in these pages is intended to improve the strength and shape of your upper body and to provide advice and tips that you can actually use in the gym to enhance your training. It's information that can be put into action immediately. We're direct with every topic yet thorough enough in our explanations so that you are not left asking further questions. Our overriding goal is that after reading this book you can go straight to the gym without having to refer to any other resource.

Because we want to present the information in a concise package, we've kept the breadth of information focused. This is why only the arms and upper body are covered in this book. It's not that working the legs isn't important—it most certainly is, because training the entire body (both above and below the belt) promotes overall balance and maximizes your ability to burn calories and keep your metabolism high in order to fend off unwanted weight gain and maintain a healthy physique. But perhaps you need a little extra help with your upper body—maybe your arms aren't as big and defined as you'd like them to be, your chest or back lacks size and shape, your shoulders don't fill out your shirts, or all of these are issues you need to work on.

One thing this manual will help with is in developing a better-looking upper body. There are undeniable health benefits to this, but if looking in the mirror to see a more appealing chest, shoulders, back, and arms is what you're after, this book is for you.

In the spirit of being easy to follow for just about anyone, this manual progresses logically so that it starts out basic and gets more advanced the further you get into it. Chapter 1 lays the groundwork for everything to follow by covering the basic muscular anatomy of the chest, back, shoulders, and arms. As you'll notice, this is not simply an Anatomy 101 course. Rather, it's applied anatomy, meaning we tell you exactly how knowing the specifics of your upper-body musculature will affect your training in the gym. You'll be able to target specific areas of each muscle to improve on weak areas in your physique, such as a narrow back, a scrawny upper chest, or biceps that lack a peak.

Our objective is to not spend any more time than is absolutely necessary on the most basic material. We want to get you to the advanced material as soon as possible. Thus, chapter 2 builds on the anatomy primer with training parameters that provide a solid foundation from which all of your training will stem, regardless of your level of expertise. Recommended frequency of training is explained in detail, as are the number of sets to perform per muscle group in each workout, the intensity at which you should train, and advice on adding variety into your program for continued success.

Chapter 3 advances the training guidelines even further by taking the discussion into greater detail. The topics discussed include the repetition ranges that work best for muscular size, strength, and endurance; recommended rest periods between sets; speed of reps (from slow reps to explosive training); the types of exercises that you can perform (compound and isolation movements); and advice on organizing an appropriate weekly training split.

The distinguishing feature of chapters 2 and 3 (as well as subsequent chapters in the book) is that each topic of discussion takes into account multiple training goals. We realize that not every person has the same objective. One person's priority might be to add size, whereas someone else might want to maintain muscle mass but lose body fat to get leaner and more defined. Another person's goal might be to improve muscular strength and power to improve performance in sports. All of these major goals are covered, and within each topic in chapters 2 and 3, we even address those who are looking for a little of everything. The knowledge you gain here will allow you to confidently design your own training program. And that's just part I of the book.

Part II (chapters 4 through 9) focuses on specific exercises and presents more than 100 exercises to help you reach your goals. The reason we've included such a large number of exercises is to promote variety in your weightlifting program. Performing the same exercises over an extended period of time allows muscles to adapt to the redundancy of the movements and, as a result, increases in muscular size and strength diminish. Even seemingly minor variations in an exercise (changing the bench angle slightly or using dumbbells or cables instead of a barbell) will create a new stimulus for the muscles.

Each chapter in part II includes exercise photos and descriptions explaining how to perform each exercise for the muscle group (chest, back, shoulders, triceps, biceps, forearms, and rotator cuff) highlighted in that chapter. The exact movement of each exercise is detailed in start and execution descriptions. The start descriptions explain how to prepare to do the exercise and the starting point for each rep. The execution descriptions explain how to perform a complete rep of the exercise, including the concentric and eccentric portions and what defines full range of motion.

Each exercise also details the target (the muscle the exercise emphasizes—not every muscle involved in the movement), when to perform the exercise during your workout (early on, in the middle, or toward the end of the training session), variations of the same movement (seated and standing, various hand placements), advanced tips to increase the difficulty and effectiveness of the exercise, and a list of substitutions that train the muscle group in nearly the same plane or angle. The substitutes can be used interchangeably with the original exercise to increase variety or suit individual preferences. Very few training books include such thorough information for every exercise.

Part III (chapters 10 through 12) caters to experienced lifters. The advanced training methods in chapter 10 take you through the most intense techniques that elite athletes use today—such practices as supersets, drop sets, rest-pauses, forced reps, partial reps, and negatives. A full description of each technique is followed by examples of how to incorporate the method into your training. Adding intensity to your program via such techniques will help you break through training plateaus to experience continued gains in muscular size, strength, and definition.

Chapter 11 takes all the information covered in the first 10 chapters and incorporates it into three separate three-month training programs, one for each of the major goals addressed in this book: size, strength, and fat burning. We have a very specific reason for providing these programs. Most training books give you the information on building your own program (which is presented in part I) but won't take the extra step of actually designing one for you. Here, we give you the option of either designing your own program or using one of ours, which takes all the guesswork out of the equation.

As with chapter 11, in chapter 12 the work is done for you. Chapter 12 provides individual workouts (dozens of them, in fact) because many experienced lifters are satisfied with their current programs and don't wish to abandon them in favor of a completely new one. But most people do wish to work in a novel routine from time to time to stimulate the body in a different way. When your training sessions begin to get monotonous and lose their effectiveness, sometimes all it takes to get things back on track is a fresh workout, even if just for one day.

You can incorporate the workouts in chapter 12 into your current program as you wish without throwing you off schedule. Each routine addresses a unique goal, including improving on a weak area of a particular muscle group, burning maximum calories and body fat in a given workout, and saving time in the gym for days when work or family prevents you from spending more than 30 minutes working out.

From start to finish, this book fills a major void in the genre of training and fitness books: that of an easy-to-navigate, reader-friendly guide that's focused on the areas of the body that you most want to develop—*the arms and upper body*. Your time is precious, and you have only so much of it to dedicate to reading a book about weightlifting. Moreover, you're better off going to the gym than you are reading about it. *Stronger Arms & Upper Body* will help you get the results you want by getting you to the gym more quickly and by giving you the information you need in order to improve your workouts.

Exercise Finder

	MUSCLE TRAINING TARGETS					
	CHEST					
Exercises	**Upper pectorals**	**Middle pectorals**	**Lower pectorals**	**Outer pectorals**	**Inner pectorals**	**Page**
Barbell bench press		✓				**45**
Smith machine bench press		✓				**46**
Machine press		✓				**47**
Push-up		✓				**48**
Dumbbell press —flat bench		✓				**49**
Dumbbell fly— flat bench		✓		✓		**50**
Cable fly		✓		✓	✓	**51**
Machine fly				✓	✓	**52**
Exercise ball dumbbell press —advanced*		✓				**53**
Exercise ball dumbbell fly— advanced*		✓		✓		**54**
Assisted dip— machine		✓	✓			**55**
Dip—wide grip		✓	✓			**56**
Dumbbell pull- over		✓	✓			**57**
Incline barbell press	✓					**58**
Incline dumbbell press	✓					**59**
Incline dumbbell fly	✓			✓		**60**
Decline barbell press			✓			**61**
Decline dumbbell press			✓			**62**

*Exercises that also train core and stabilizing muscles.

(continued)

Exercises	Upper pectorals	Middle pectorals	Lower pectorals	Outer pectorals	Inner pectorals	Page
Decline dumbbell fly			✓	✓		63
Cable crossover			✓	✓	✓	64

BACK

Exercises	Upper latissimus muscles	Lower latissimus muscles	Rhom-boids	Middle trapezius	Lower back	Page
Lat pull-down	✓					67
Pull-up — wide grip	✓					68
Assisted pull-up	✓					69
Lat pull-down— reverse grip		✓				70
Pull-up— close grip		✓				71
Straight-arm cable pull-down		✓				72
Dumbell straight-arm pull-back		✓				73
Barbell bent-over row		✓	✓	✓		74
Smith machine bent-over row		✓	✓	✓		75
Dumbbell bent-over row		✓	✓	✓		76
One-arm dumbbell row		✓	✓	✓		77
Smith machine one-arm row		✓	✓	✓		78
Incline dumbbell row		✓	✓	✓		79
Seated cable row		✓	✓	✓		80
Low pulley one-arm cable row		✓	✓	✓		81
T-bar row		✓	✓	✓		82
Supported t-bar row		✓	✓	✓		83

Exercises	Upper latissimus muscles	Lower latissimus muscles	Rhomboids	Middle trapezius	Lower back	Page
Machine row		✓	✓	✓		84
Back extension					✓	85
Back extension machine					✓	86
Lying back extension					✓	87

SHOULDERS AND TRAPEZIUS

Exercises	Front deltoids	Middle deltoids	Rear deltoids	Upper trapezius	Middle trapezius	Page
Barbell overhead press	✓	✓				91
Dumbbell overhead press	✓	✓				92
Smith machine overhead press	✓	✓				93
Machine overhead press	✓	✓				94
Barbell upright row	✓	✓		✓		95
Dumbbell upright row	✓	✓		✓		96
Cable upright row	✓	✓		✓		97
Smith machine upright row	✓	✓		✓		98
Arnold press	✓	✓				99
Dumbbell lateral raise		✓				100
Cable lateral raise		✓				101
Machine lateral raise		✓				102
Dumbbell front raise	✓					103
Barbell front raise	✓					104
Incline barbell front raise	✓					105

(continued)

Exercises	Front deltoids	Middle deltoids	Rear deltoids	Upper trapezius	Middle trapezius	Page
Prone incline barbell front raise	✓					106
Cable front raise	✓					107
Dumbbell bent-over lateral raise			✓			108
Cable bent-over lateral raise			✓			109
Cable reverse fly			✓			110
Machine reverse fly			✓			111
Cross-body rear deltoid raise			✓			112
Barbell shrug				✓		113
Dumbbell shrug				✓		114
Smith machine shrug				✓		115
Cable shrug				✓		116
Prone incline dumbbell shrug				✓	✓	117

TRICEPS

Exercises	Triceps lateral head	Triceps long head	Triceps medial head	Page
Barbell bench press—close grip	✓			121
Smith machine bench press—close grip	✓			122
Push-up—narrow hand position	✓			123
Cable press-down	✓			124
Dumbbell kickback	✓			125
Cable kickback	✓			126

Exercises	Triceps lateral head	Triceps long head	Triceps medial head	Page
Decline lying barbell extension	✓			127
Lying barbell extension	✓	✓		128
Lying dumbbell extension	✓	✓		129
Lying cable extension	✓	✓		130
Dip—narrow grip	✓		✓	131
Bench dip	✓		✓	132
Dumbbell overhead extension		✓		133
Barbell overhead extension		✓		134
Cable overhead extension		✓		135
Seated overhead cable extension		✓		136
Smith machine overhead extension		✓		137
Barbell bench press—reverse grip			✓	138
Cable press-down —reverse grip			✓	139

BICEPS AND FOREARMS

Exercises	Biceps long head	Biceps short head	Brachialis	Brachio-radialis	Forearms	Page
Barbell curl	✓	✓				143
Alternating dumbbell curl	✓	✓				144
Seated barbell curl	✓	✓				145
Cable curl	✓	✓				146

(continued)

Exercises	Biceps long head	Biceps short head	Brachialis	Brachio-radialis	Forearms	Page
Drag curl	✓	✓				147
Incline cable curl	✓	✓				148
Incline dumbbell curl	✓					149
Concentration curl	✓					150
Cable con-centration curl	✓					151
Lying cable con-centration curl		✓				152
Barbell preacher curl		✓				153
Dumbbell preacher curl		✓				154
Cable preacher curl		✓				155
Machine preacher curl		✓				156
High cable curl		✓				157
Hammer curl	✓		✓			158
Cable hammer curl	✓		✓			159
Barbell reverse curl			✓	✓		160
Dumbbell reverse curl			✓	✓		161
Cable reverse curl			✓	✓		162
Preacher reverse curl			✓	✓		163
Standing wrist curl					✓	164
Seated wrist curl					✓	165
Behind-the-back wrist curl					✓	166
Standing reverse wrist curl					✓	167

ROTATOR CUFF					
Exercises	Supra-spinatus	Infraspinatus	Teres minor	Sub-scapularis	Page
Dumbbell external rotation		✓	✓		171
Three-way raise	✓	✓	✓		172
Cable or elastic band external rotation		✓	✓		174
Dumbbell internal rotation				✓	175
Cable or elastic band internal rotation				✓	176
Empty can	✓				177

PART I

Foundations to Training

CHAPTER 1

Upper-Body Anatomy

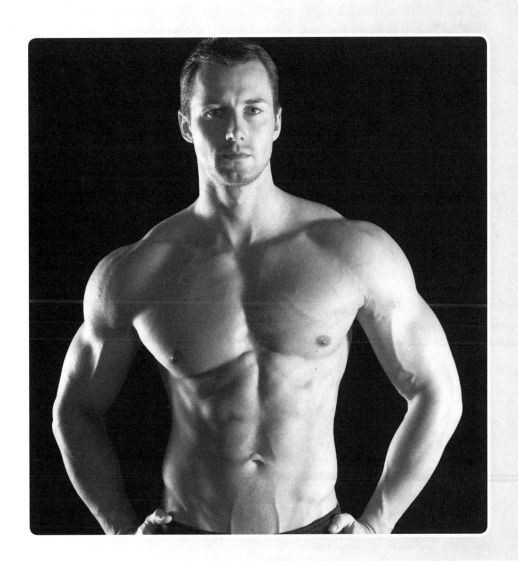

All the muscles of the upper body—those of the chest, back, shoulders, and arms—work together in daily activities, athletic movements, and full-body lifting exercises. Opposing muscle groups (chest and back, biceps and triceps) balance each other out and provide stability while the other is contracting. But in traditional weight training, individual muscles are isolated as a means of overloading specific areas and developing the musculature of the entire body to its potential. This is why, in discussions of the anatomy of the upper body and how it pertains to your training, each of the major muscle groups is addressed separately, despite the fact that in the end they'll all be working as a group.

This chapter provides an overview of the muscles of the chest, back, shoulders, arms, and rotator cuff. For each, the names and locations of the major individual muscles are discussed as well as the anatomical movements they initiate and how you can target specific areas of each muscle group in your training. As you'll notice, each muscle group is composed of either multiple muscles or multiple heads of a particular muscle, and often times both. Achieving full development in muscular size and strength, as well as overall muscular balance, requires training each individual muscle as well as specific areas of individual muscles. This chapter provides you with a working knowledge of the anatomy of the upper body, which lays the foundation for all the training techniques, both basic and advanced, and specifics on program design found throughout this book.

CHEST

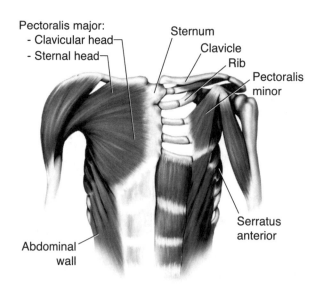

The primary muscles of the chest.

Muscles Involved

The primary muscle that makes up the chest is the pectoralis major (sometimes called pecs or pectorals). It spans from the clavicle down to the upper abdominal wall and from the sternum out laterally across the shoulder on either side (each side, to the right and left of the sternum, makes up one muscle). Pectoralis major is composed of two heads: the clavicular head, comprising the upper borders of the pectorals, and the considerably larger sternal head, which spans the middle and lower portions of the chest.

Pectoralis minor (which, despite its name, does not actually assist pectoralis major) lies underneath pectoralis major, attaching from the third, fourth, and fifth ribs up to the scapula on either side. The fingerlike serratus anterior resides laterally and below the pectorals on either side (attached to the ribs) and is involved in many of the same movements as pectoralis major and minor are.

Target Training

Many people find that their upper pectorals (the clavicular head) lack the size and thickness of the middle and lower pectorals (sternal head). Targeting the upper pectorals to increase the size is a matter of performing any type of pressing or fly exercise on an inclined bench at an angle of 30 to 45 degrees. Recent physiological studies have also shown that doing barbell pressing exercises with a reverse (underhand) grip, as well as dumbbell presses with a neutral grip, targets the upper pectorals. Cable crossovers performed with the line of pull coming from low pulleys to up in front of the chest trains the upper pectorals as well. (See chapter 4 for descriptions, photos, and advice on chest exercises.)

The entire sternal head of the pectorals is trained during presses and fly exercises on a flat bench as well as with cable crossovers in which the pulleys are positioned at a high to medium height and the handles are pulled out in front of the chest. And since the sternal head is significantly larger than the clavicle head, exercises on the flat bench are ideal for building size and strength because more weight can be used.

You can target the lower portion of the sternal head, just above where the abdominal wall begins, by performing presses and flys on a decline bench set at a 15- to 45-degree angle (that is, the shoulders are below the level of the hips). Additionally, cable crossovers in which the pulleys are set high and the handles are pulled together down below the waist emphasize the lower pectorals. Focusing on such exercises can be especially helpful if you lack thickness in the lower chest.

Creating width in the chest by developing the outer portions of the pectorals, as well as achieving separation between the right and left pectoral muscles by targeting the inner pectorals, is important if you're looking to achieve a well-shaped chest rather than size alone. The outer and inner pectorals (both heads) are emphasized during fly and crossover exercises in which the arms remain in an extended position throughout. The inner pectorals are especially emphasized at the top of the movement, where the hands come together and the pectorals can be squeezed to intensify the contraction. The outer pectorals are also emphasized when using a wide grip (outside shoulder width) on barbell presses, and the inner pectorals are stressed to a greater degree with a grip just inside shoulder width. You can target the serratus and pectoralis minor by extending the range of motion on presses at the top by allowing your shoulders to come off the bench as you push the bar or dumbbells as high as possible over you.

BACK

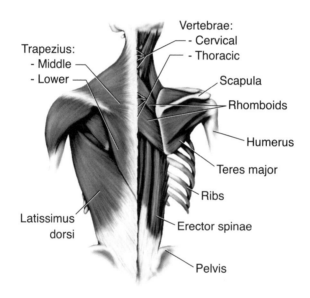

The primary muscles of the back.

Muscles Involved

The major muscles of the back are the latissimus dorsi (the largest muscle and often called lats), teres major, middle and lower trapezius, rhomboids, and erector spinae (lower back). (A myriad of other smaller muscles are present as well, but they are not the focus here.) The latissimus dorsi extends from the pelvis, vertebral column, and ribs all the way up to the humerus (upper arm bone) on either side. The teres major, a relatively small muscle, originates from the scapula and also connects to the humerus.

These two muscles, particularly the latissimus dorsi, produce the width of the back.

The middle and lower trapezius and rhomboids make up the thickness of the middle back because both attach from the upper vertebrae to the scapulae on either side; the rhomboids lie beneath the trapezius, and thus are less visible to the naked eye. The erector spinae muscles actually run along the entire length of the back (from the pelvis up to the cervical vertebrae of the neck), though they lie beneath other major back muscles and are only visible in the lower region.

Target Training

The simplest way to distinguish between back exercises is to separate them into two groups: those that increase back width and those that add thickness. Pull-downs and pull-ups emphasize the latissimus dorsi and teres major and thus are ideal for creating width. Rowing exercises, while also hitting the latissimus dorsi, rely to a greater degree on the middle-back muscles (rhomboids and middle and lower trapezius) and will add thickness. Each back workout you do should consist of both pull-down and pull-up movements and rows, though the ratio and order in which they're performed should differ depending on whether you lack width or thickness in the back. (Prioritizing is discussed further in chapter 3.)

You can target areas of the latissimus dorsi with specific exercises as well as with varying hand positions on similar movements. Taking a wide (outside shoulder width) overhand grip on lat pull-downs and pull-ups emphasizes the fibers of the upper latissimus muscles as well as the teres major. Conversely, assuming a narrow (inside shoulder width) reverse grip or neutral grip trains the lower latissimus dorsi to a greater extent. If you want to add overall back width, use wide-grip variations.

Even on rowing exercises (cable rows, T-bar rows, and even bent-over barbell rows), taking a wide grip (again, outside shoulder width) and pulling the bar or handle to a higher point on your chest targets the upper latissimus muscles while also training the rhomboids and middle trapezius. Using a narrow grip (the hands shoulder width or closer), especially when using a reverse grip and pulling the bar or handle to your lower abdominals, emphasizes the lower latissimus dorsi. Because the rhomboids and middle trapezius are smaller than the latissimus muscles, targeting different areas of them would be marginally noticeable at best. However, pulling the bar to a higher point, as in the previous example, requires greater involvement of the middle trapezius and rhomboids.

Targeting the lower back is simply a matter of performing back extension exercises that isolate the erector spinae muscles. Emphasizing specific areas of the lower back is largely unnecessary. (Descriptions, photos, and advice on back exercises are in chapter 5.)

SHOULDERS AND UPPER TRAPEZIUS

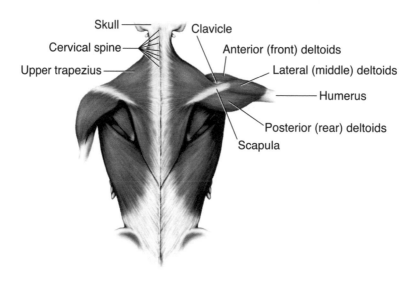

The primary muscles of the shoulders.

Muscles Involved

Three muscles make up the shoulders: the anterior (front) deltoids, middle (lateral) deltoids, and posterior (rear) deltoids. These three muscles (also called delts) wrap around each shoulder from front to back. The anterior deltoids originate from the clavicle, the middle and posterior deltoids originate from different points on the scapula, and all insert at the same point on the humerus (upper arm bone).

When someone mentions the "traps," typically he or she is referring to the upper trapezius muscles, as opposed to the middle or lower trapezius that are more often considered part of the back musculature. The upper trapezius muscles are located on top of the shoulders, attaching from the skull and cervical spine to the clavicle on either side. Unlike the middle or lower trapezius, the upper trapezius can be seen from the front as well as from the back and side, which is why they're often classified as shoulder muscles.

Target Training

It's common to have an imbalance among the three deltoid muscles. The anterior deltoids are often overdeveloped because of their constant involvement in chest exercises. If that's the case for you, focus on the middle and posterior deltoids when training the shoulders to minimize deltoid imbalances that could lead to injury. Emphasizing one deltoid muscle over another is a simple matter of performing the lateral raise variation specific to the deltoid you want to target. Front raises isolate the anterior deltoids, lateral raises focus on the middle deltoids, and bent-over raises target the posterior deltoids. In the previous example, where the anterior deltoids overpower the other two deltoids, forgoing front raises in favor of lateral and bent-over laterals is wise.

Compound exercises for the shoulders (overhead press and upright row) don't specifically isolate any one of the deltoids. Although the middle deltoids are involved in all overhead presses and upright rows, doing presses behind the neck emphasizes them more; presses in front of the head involve the front deltoids more. Upright rows, which are always performed in front of the body, engage the front deltoids along with the middle deltoids and deemphasize the posterior deltoids.

The upper trapezius muscles are involved in virtually every shoulder exercise because the shoulders are elevated to some degree on every rep of overhead presses, upright rows, and front and lateral raises. However, rarely is a full range of motion achieved by the upper trapezius during these exercises. The only way to truly isolate the trapezius from the three deltoid muscles is to perform barbell, dumbbell, or machine shrugs, thereby deactivating the movement at the shoulder joint and performing only shoulder girdle elevation through a full range of motion. Include shrugs in your shoulder routine not only to improve weak upper trapezius muscles but to promote balance in the shoulder region as a whole.

TRICEPS

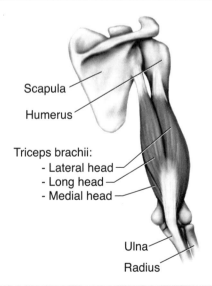

Scapula

Humerus

Triceps brachii:
- Lateral head
- Long head
- Medial head

Ulna

Radius

The triceps muscles.

Muscles Involved

The back of the upper arm contains just one muscle, the triceps brachii, which is composed of three separate heads: lateral head, medial head, and long head. The long head originates at the scapula; the other two heads arise from the humerus on either side. All three heads insert at the ulna (the forearm bone on the pinky-finger side).

Target Training

Fully developed triceps bulge out to the side where the lateral head is prominent, are thick and defined in the inner portion because of the medial head, and are the most massive up near the shoulder, which is where the long head resides. If any of these areas is deficient, you can target the lateral, medial, or long head by altering the position of the arms. However, keep in mind that any time the elbow is extended, all three heads of the triceps work together to initiate the movement; it's virtually impossible to isolate any one head completely. The lateral head is targeted during close-grip bench presses; standard cable press-downs also place slightly more emphasis on the lateral head than the other two. The medial head is emphasized when using a reverse grip, as when doing the reverse-grip version of press-downs, bench presses, or lying extensions. Triceps exercises in which the arms are overhead (all variations of overhead extensions) target the long head.

BICEPS AND FOREARMS

Muscles Involved

The muscles of the upper anterior arm are the biceps brachii and the smaller brachialis. The biceps brachii is made up of the long (outer) head and short (inner) head. Both heads attach from the scapula to the radius and ulna (the two forearm bones). The brachialis, which runs below the biceps brachii, originates from the humerus and crosses the elbow joint to attach to the ulna.

The forearms are composed of many relatively small muscles; the major one is the brachioradialis and the others are typically referred to collectively as either wrist flexors or wrist extensors. (Each forearm muscle does in fact have a distinct name, but for simplicity's sake we use these broad categories; "wrist flexors" refers to the anterior forearm muscles and "wrist extensors" to the posterior forearm muscles.) The brachioradialis attaches from the humerus to the radius, and the wrist flexors and extensors originate at various points on the humerus, radius, and ulna (the flexors on the palm side of the forearm and the extensors on the opposite side) and cross the wrist joint to attach to various areas on the hand.

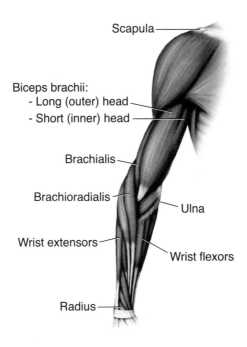

Scapula

Biceps brachii:
- Long (outer) head
- Short (inner) head

Brachialis

Brachioradialis

Ulna

Wrist extensors

Wrist flexors

Radius

The biceps and forearm muscles.

Target Training

Because the long head of the biceps is located outside of the short head, using a narrow grip (inside shoulder width) when doing barbell curls emphasizes development of the long head. Taking a grip that is outside shoulder width, on the other hand, will target the short head. The long head, which makes up the much-desired portion of the biceps often referred to as the peak, is also targeted during hammer curls, in which the wrists don't supinate during the movement and the palms face each other throughout.

Developing the brachialis muscles can maximize thickness in the upper arms. Since it plays a role in elbow flexion and no part in forearm supination (rotating the forearms from a palms down to palms up position), isolating the brachialis is a matter of doing hammer curls. The brachioradialis provides thickness to the thumb side of the upper forearms, an area in which many people lack size. Like the brachialis, the brachioradialis has no role in wrist supination, so hammer curls target that muscle. So do reverse curls, in which the bar is gripped with the palms down so that the forearms are in a fully pronated position (the opposite of supinated) throughout the exercise.

The forearm flexors and extensors are small enough that attempting to target a specific area of either muscle would be hardly noticeable. Simply doing wrist curls for the flexors and reverse wrist curls for the extensors isolates each sufficiently.

ROTATOR CUFF

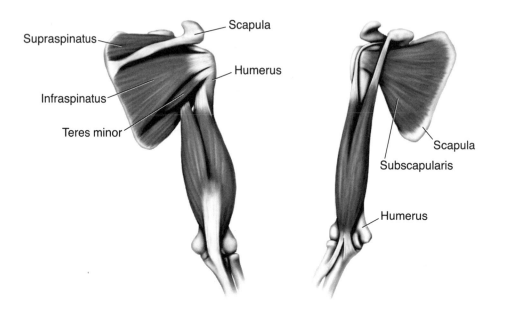

Anterior and posterior views of the shoulder reveal the rotator cuff muscles.

Muscles Involved

The muscles of the rotator cuff are the supraspinatus, infraspinatus, teres minor, and subscapularis (the acronym SITS for short). Each of the four small SITS muscles originates from a distinct point on the scapula and inserts on the upper portion of the humerus on either side.

Target Training

Even though the SITS muscles contract during chest, shoulder, and back exercises, they must be isolated separately in order to be strengthened. In fact, it's because they're so involved in stabilizing the shoulders during other upper-body exercises that conditioning them is so vital; overloading them with hundreds of pounds when doing chest and shoulder presses and pull-downs and rows for the back can lead to tearing of these relatively tiny muscles if they're not properly strengthened. The bottom line is that training the SITS muscles is not about enhancing their appearance; rather, it's about preventing injury, specifically muscle tears in the rotator cuff that require surgery and months of time away from the gym.

Exercises that isolate the rotator cuff muscles are subtle movements that you should perform with very light weight (relative to your strength) because overloading these muscles with heavy resistance while isolating them can lead to injury. Furthermore, never perform rotator cuff exercises to muscular failure. (See chapter 9 for more information on rotator cuff exercises.)

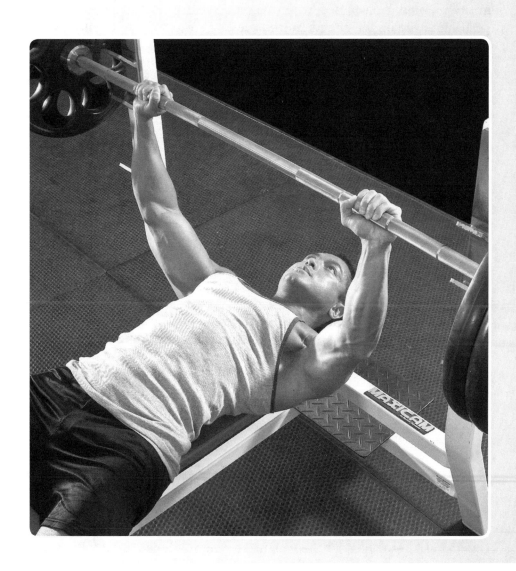

CHAPTER 2

Training Fundamentals

This book is by no means for beginning lifters only. The chapters that follow address the most advanced, cutting-edge training concepts that exercise science has to offer. But laying a foundation of basics is in order both for novice lifters who are getting up to speed and for experienced lifters who could use a refresher on the basics. This chapter provides the fundamental training concepts that anyone who trains with weights should know, beginning with a quick review of the basic grips for weightlifting.

As you work your way through the individual muscle groups and exercises throughout this book, you'll find information about the effects of changing your grip position. Changing the grip on an exercise works the muscle from a slightly different angle, which targets a different area of the muscle than the standard grip for that exercise. Grip variations are most commonly discussed when using a barbell, but changes in hand position have similar effects on muscles when using dumbbells, cables, and various machines.

Three basic types of grips are used in weightlifting: pronated, supinated, and neutral. With a pronated grip, often called overhand, you hold the weight with your forearms in a pronated position (rotated so that the thumbs point inward), but the direction the palms and forearms face varies. When using a pronated grip on lat pull-downs, for example, the palms and forearms face forward. However, when using a pronated grip on barbell curls (reverse curl), the palms and forearms face behind you at the start of each rep, then face forward by the top of the rep. With a supinated, or underhand, grip, you rotate the forearms so that the thumbs point outward and keep them in that position as you perform a given exercise. When doing a lat pull-down with a supinated grip (reverse-grip pull-down), for example, your palms and forearms face behind you. Likewise, when doing a reverse-grip bench press, your palms and forearms face in the direction of your head. With a neutral grip, the palms and forearms face toward each other as when doing hammer curls.

The term *reverse grip*, which is used throughout this book, simply refers to whatever grip position is the opposite of the standard grip for a given exercise. A reverse grip usually refers to a supinated (underhand) grip, but not always. A reverse-grip bench press and a reverse-grip lat pull-down, for example, require a supinated grip because the standard grip for those exercises is pronated. However, a reverse curl requires a pronated grip because the standard grip for this exercise is supinated.

INTENSITY (TRAINING TO FAILURE)

The term *intensity* is used in various contexts when it comes to lifting weights. Many people use the word simply to express how much weight is being used—the heavier the weight, the more intense the set. But that's only half the equation. Intensity is actually the amount of weight used in a given set plus the number of repetitions that are performed with that weight. The intensity of a set is relative to each person; a set of 10 reps with 80 pounds will be very intense for some people yet very easy (not so intense) for others. Conversions of pounds to kilograms are included in the appendix on page 241.

To simplify things further, intensity can be equated with the concept of training to failure, which means doing a set with a given weight to the point at which one more rep with that weight on your own is physically impossible. For instance, if the most reps you can do with 80 pounds is 10, and you did 10 reps, you trained to failure on that set; if you stopped after 8 reps, you didn't train to failure. (Chapter 10 discusses advanced techniques that allow you to train past failure to further increase intensity.) Therefore, intensity isn't simply a matter of how much weight you use or how many reps you do but rather whether you trained to failure. A set of 20 reps can be just as intense as a set of 6 reps, even if you used a significantly lighter weight, provided you took that set to failure (you weren't able to do a 21st rep).

Training to failure is a double-edged sword. On one hand, the only way to truly maximize your potential for muscle growth and strength is to take sets to failure. At the same time, however, training to failure too often can lead to overtraining. To avoid overtraining, don't train to failure on more than one or two sets per exercise. For example, you might plan to do three sets of 8 to 12 reps on barbell curls. In the first set, maybe you can do 12 reps maximum. Instead of doing 12, do 10. In the next set, using the same weight, maybe 11 reps is all you can do. Again, do 10. In your last set, do as many reps as you possibly can, whether that ends up being 8, 9, or 10. Just make sure you don't have even one more rep in you. You can then move on to your next exercise having gotten the most out of your three sets of curls while not overdoing it.

VOLUME

Volume refers to the total amount of work performed. Many strength coaches and trainers use the number of sets, the reps performed in each set, and the amount of weight per set in describing volume; however, for simplicity's sake, volume is defined here as the total number of working sets (not including warm-up sets) performed in a given workout and, more specifically, for a particular muscle group. How much volume you should train with depends on your goals (see table 2.1):

■ **Size.** If you want to increase the size of your muscles (that is, hypertrophy), employ high-volume training—9 to 20 sets per workout for larger

TABLE 2.1   **Suggested Total Number of Sets per Week**

Goal	Chest, back, shoulders	Biceps, triceps, trapezius, forearms
Muscular size	9-20	6-16
Muscular strength and power	9-16	6-12
Muscular definition	12-20	9-16

muscle groups (chest, back, and shoulders) and roughly 6 to 16 sets for smaller muscle groups (triceps, biceps, trapezius, and forearms). These ranges are somewhat broad, but most exercise scientists versed in hypertrophy training agree with these parameters because they've been supported through both formal research and anecdotal observations (that is, people who have tried these methods in the gym and then reported their experiences).

The reason for training larger muscle groups with higher volume is that a larger muscle (which contains a greater number of muscle fibers) requires a greater stimulus to grow than a smaller muscle requires. Moreover, smaller body parts are also trained when larger muscle groups are working. For example, when you're doing a pressing exercise for the chest, your shoulders and triceps are also helping perform the movement, even though they're not the primary movers; likewise, your biceps are working when you perform rows, pull-downs, and pull-ups for the back. Because of this, smaller muscle groups will require less volume when you train them specifically.

■ **Strength.** Powerlifters, whose sole objective is to gain strength, typically perform significantly fewer total sets than those whose main goal is to add size. The reason is that as the number of sets in a given workout increases, strength and power levels decrease. When strength levels are diminished, a powerlifter has little use for further training and is better off stopping to allow his muscles to recover so he can be strong for the next lifting session. When all-out strength is your goal, keep your total number of sets moderate: 9 to 16 sets for large muscle groups per workout and 6 to 12 sets for smaller ones.

■ **Muscular definition.** People typically differentiate muscular size from muscular definition, as if there's a distinct way to go about attaining each. However, when muscles grow via high-volume weight training, the body's metabolism increases because muscle is metabolically active tissue. When your metabolism increases, you burn more fat and become leaner, thereby increasing muscular definition. Therefore, to increase definition, you should train with the same volume as you would when training for size. Nearly every competitive bodybuilder, whose goal is to get bigger and more defined, trains with high volume. However, unlike bodybuilders, many people have a goal of improving definition without experiencing a considerable increase in size of muscles. Achieving this is more a matter of the amount of weight you use, the number of reps you do per set, and your training frequency than it is a matter of volume.

TRAINING FREQUENCY

Training frequency refers to how many times per week you train each muscle group. Regardless of whether you choose once, twice, or three times per week, the weekly volume will remain the same (9 to 20 sets for larger body parts, 6 to 16 for smaller ones), but you can divide the volume for each workout by 2 if you're training each body part twice per week and by 3 for training three times per week. For example, if you decide to train the chest just one time per week, you would do all 9 to 20 sets that day. On the other hand, people who train each muscle group more frequently (two or three times per week) generally train with less volume per workout. It all comes down to recovery—making sure your muscles are sufficiently rested before you train them again.

Unfortunately, we can't tell you how much rest you'll need between workouts for each body part; that is something you'll find out as you gain more experience. Some people judge their readiness by muscle soreness: If a muscle is still sore from the previous workout, hold off on training it again until it's pain free. But this is not a foolproof method of determining a muscle's recovery status because an experienced lifter might be sore for only two days after a 16-set chest workout even though his muscles are still not sufficiently recovered for another few days after that. Soreness alone is not an adequate indicator.

When deciding what frequency is best for you, start with your goal. If strength is your main objective, train each muscle group once or twice per week. The reason is that you want your muscles fully rested each time you train, and you'll want to give your full attention to each body part, knowing you won't have to train it again a couple days later.

If building size (hypertrophy) is your goal, you should train each body part either once or twice per week as well. The reasoning is similar to that for gaining strength—to give each muscle group your undivided attention during the session and to allow for full recovery after the session. You'll find training each muscle group once or twice a week allows you to achieve this.

If your goal is to lose a significant amount of body fat, train each body part three times per week. If you go to the gym three days a week, you'll be training all muscle groups in each workout, doing a full-body routine. Because you're working your entire body every time you train, you'll tend to burn more calories. Chapter 3 goes into more depth about prioritizing your training according to your goals as well as your strengths and weaknesses.

VARIETY

Changing things up is a key training concept when it comes to maximizing your muscles' potential to grow bigger and stronger over the long term. Promoting variety in your weightlifting program is one of the best ways to ensure you won't waste your time and get stuck at lifting plateaus in which you see very little results for long periods.

Your body will adapt to anything it's asked to do on a repeated basis. Likewise, any new stimulus you throw at it will elicit a change. So you need to constantly change your workouts. As a general rule, do not do the same workout for more than eight consecutive weeks. To that end, here are the major variables that you can change in your routine on a regular basis:

■ **Exercises.** Don't do the exact same exercises day in and day out. If on the last day that you trained your chest you did barbell bench presses, next time substitute dumbbell presses or machine presses. For the back, alternate between lat pull-downs and pull-ups, or do bent-over barbell rows instead of cable rows. The possibilities are endless; you can substitute numerous exercises, many of which are in chapters 4 to 9.

■ **Exercise order.** Another way to add variety is to change the order in which you do the exercises. If, in your previous chest workout, you did flat bench presses first and incline presses second, do incline presses first the next time around. If you always do cable press-downs for triceps before all other triceps moves, try doing it last occasionally. This is a particularly good way to add variety when exercise choices are limited, such as for those who train at home.

■ **Sets, reps, and resistance.** Don't always stick to three sets of 10 reps or four sets of 8 reps on every exercise. Mix in high volume (five or six sets for an exercise) with low volume (two or three sets) and high reps (15 to 20) with low reps (5 or 6). Chapter 3 covers these variables in greater depth.

■ **Rest periods.** How long you rest between sets should change on a regular basis and depends on your goal. But in terms of variety, don't always rest 1 minute between sets, for example. Experiment with shorter rest periods (30 to 45 seconds) and longer ones (2 to 3 minutes) to see how your muscles respond and recover.

These are just a handful of ways to add variety to your training to keep your muscles from adapting and your results from becoming stagnant.

Another way to make sure your training is constantly changing is to do a periodized program that consists of different phases, or cycles, over the course of a few months or even a year or more. The phases typically alter volume, rep ranges, rest between sets, and exercise selection to help you achieve various goals throughout the course of the program, even if you have one overriding objective in mind (such as strength, size, or definition). Examples of periodized programs that manipulate all of the training variables are presented in chapter 11.

OVERTRAINING

Overtraining is a simple concept: It occurs when you train too much, to the point at which your efforts not only fail to produce positive results but are actually counterproductive. Doing too much volume in the gym can make you weaker, compromise your immune system, and make you more injury prone because muscles, ligaments, and tendons can become strained, sprained, or even torn when overloaded in a fatigued state. Furthermore, training with too much volume suppresses levels of the anabolic (muscle-building) hormones testosterone and growth hormone (GH) in your body and increases levels of the hormone cortisol, which in high amounts causes muscle wasting. It's extremely important to keep these hormones at their optimal levels (testosterone and GH high, cortisol low) to maximize your efforts in the gym.

With respect to upper-body training, there are several commonly overtrained areas. The shoulders are one, since the deltoid muscles are worked when you train both your chest and back. If you train each muscle group once a week, you're essentially working your shoulders three times—in your chest workout, back workout, and shoulder workout. Because of this, you might want to train your shoulders less frequently than your chest and back or train them just as frequently but with less volume. The key is to make sure they're sufficiently rested before you train them. Chapter 3 details how to organize your training to ensure that each muscle gets proper rest.

Your rotator cuff muscles, located posteriorly on your shoulders and around your shoulder blades, are also often overworked because they serve as stabilizing muscles in many upper-body movements and end up being more fatigued than most muscle groups. The key to ensuring your rotator cuffs don't become vulnerable to injury is to do specific exercises (see chapter 9) to strengthen them so that these muscles are better conditioned to handle the enormous load placed on them as stabilizers.

"Glamour" muscle groups, such as the chest and biceps, are also commonly overtrained. Because these muscles are more visible in the mirror than the back and triceps muscles, lifters sometimes give them more attention in the gym, which creates muscular imbalances that can lead to injury. A good rule is to not train your chest with any more volume than you use to train your back, and don't train your biceps more than you train your triceps. This will promote optimal balance. Promoting muscular balance through your training split is discussed at length in chapter 3.

Every split, workout, and program presented in this book provides the optimal training stimulus for maximum results based on your goals. The objective is to neither undertrain nor overtrain your body. In addition to heeding the recommendations for volume and recovery time, getting adequate nutrition and sleep can help you avoid overtraining. Whether a muscle is overtrained depends in part on the nutrients available in the body to help repair it, including adequate amounts of protein, carbohydrate, and fat. Since this isn't a nutrition book, the topic is not covered here, but it's in your best interest to educate yourself about proper nutrition for training. Two books that can help you in this area are *Power Eating* by Susan Kleiner and Maggie Greenwood-Robinson and *Nancy Clark's Sports Nutrition Guidebook* (both are published by Human Kinetics). As for sleep, try to get seven to nine hours of sleep every night to support your efforts in the gym. Without allowing your body the rest it needs, you're undermining your training.

CHAPTER 3

Exercise Essentials

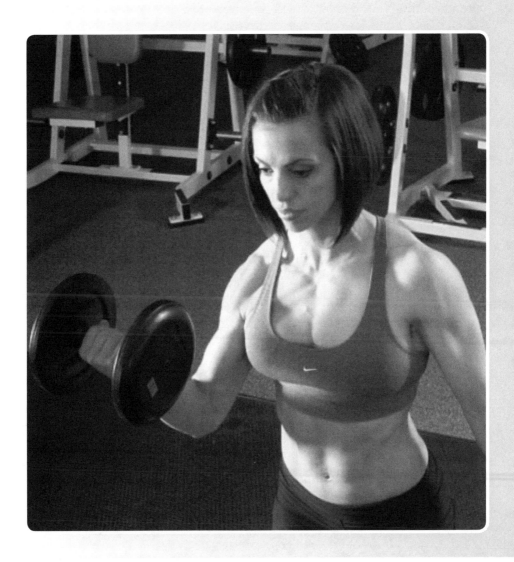

When designing a lifting program, you'll need to address several important aspects: the number of times to train per week, the types of exercises to do, the number of sets and reps to do, and the length of rest between each set. Whatever your goal, this chapter touches on all these issues and more.

TRAINING SPLIT DESIGN

A training split is simply your weekly lifting schedule—what muscle groups to train on what days. There are a myriad of ways to organize your training based on your specific goals. Consider the following aspects when creating your personalized training split:

Frequency

Start with your general training goal to determine how many times per week to train each muscle group. If strength or size is your goal, you should train each muscle group one or two times per week; three times per week for each muscle group is recommended if your goal is muscular endurance.

Types of Training Splits

After deciding on a frequency, you still have several options on arranging your training through the course of the week. These options depend on how many days per week you're willing to go to the gym, how long you want to spend lifting during each session, and which muscle groups you prefer to pair up together. Here are the most common training splits:

■ **Whole-body split** (frequency of three times per week for all muscle groups). The simplest way to train each muscle group three days a week is to go to the gym three times (Monday, Wednesday, and Friday, for example), training every muscle group in each workout. The main benefit to this is that you minimize the number of days per week you're in the gym, which works well for people who have hectic schedules and aren't able to get to the gym four to six days a week. However, training every muscle group in each workout typically means a longer training session because of greater overall volume. Keeping rest periods between sets brief, however, can speed up the workout. Table 3.1 provides an example of a basic whole-body training split.

TABLE 3.1   Whole-Body Training Split

Day	Muscle groups trained
Monday	Chest, back, shoulders, biceps, triceps, legs, abs
Tuesday	Off
Wednesday	Chest, shoulders, back, triceps, biceps, legs, abs
Thursday	Off
Friday	Legs, chest, back, shoulders, biceps, triceps, abs
Saturday	Off
Sunday	Off

■ **Two-day split** (frequency of two or three times per week for each muscle group). Another way to train each muscle group three times per week is to use a two-day split, in which you train your entire body over the course of two days, splitting the work in half so that each workout is of the same duration. This allows you to concentrate on fewer muscle groups per workout, which many people prefer, assuming you don't mind going to the gym six days a week. If strength or size is your goal and you prefer training each muscle group twice a week, the two-day split involves spending four days a week in the gym (see table 3.2).

TABLE 3.2   Standard Two-Day Split

Day	Muscle groups trained
Monday	Chest, shoulders, triceps
Tuesday	Legs, back, biceps
Wednesday	Off
Thursday	Chest, shoulders, triceps
Friday	Legs, back, biceps
Saturday	Off
Sunday	Off

How you decide to divide your muscle groups is a matter of personal preference. One way is to do an upper- and lower-body split (see table 3.3): On day 1 you train all your upper-body muscles and on day 2 all your lower-body muscles, or vice versa. Or, as shown in table 3.2, you can train both your upper- and lower-body muscles (different ones, of course) on one or both days.

TABLE 3.3   Upper- and Lower-Body Two-Day Split

Day	Muscle groups trained
Monday	Chest, back, shoulders, biceps, triceps
Tuesday	Legs
Wednesday	Off
Thursday	Chest, back, shoulders, biceps, triceps
Friday	Legs
Saturday	Off
Sunday	Off

■ **Three-day split** (frequency of one or two times per week for each muscle group). A three-day split entails training the entire body over the course of three workouts. If you want to train each muscle group once a week, you'll have a total of three workouts per week; if you want to train each muscle group twice a week, it will mean six workouts per week. One common way to divide up your training is to use the push–pull–legs split (see table 3.4): One day you'll work all of your major upper-body pushing muscle groups (chest, shoulders, triceps), another day you'll work all your upper-body pulling muscle groups (back and biceps), and the third day you'll train your legs. The main benefit to training this way is that while you're doing your pushing movements, your pulling muscles are recovering, and vice versa. Shoulders are considered a pushing muscle group despite the fact that they initiate both pushing (shoulder presses) and pulling movements (upright rows and raises). An example of a standard three-day split is provided in table 3.5.

TABLE 3.4   Push–Pull–Legs Split

Day	Muscle groups trained
Monday	Chest, shoulders, triceps
Tuesday	Back, biceps
Wednesday	Legs
Thursday	Off
Friday	Repeat Monday (optional)
Saturday	Repeat Tuesday (optional)
Sunday	Repeat Wednesday (optional)

TABLE 3.5 Standard Three-Day Split

Day	Muscle groups trained
Monday	Chest, back
Tuesday	Legs
Wednesday	Shoulders, triceps, biceps
Thursday	Off
Friday	Repeat Monday (optional)
Saturday	Repeat Tuesday (optional)
Sunday	Repeat Wednesday (optional)

■ **Four-day split** (frequency of one time per week for each muscle group). With the four-day split, you train your entire body over the course of four days. Because you're spreading your training more thinly, this split is ideal for training each muscle group once a week with high volume. With this split, you have greater flexibility with muscle pairings as well as with which days you train. For example, you can train your chest with your back, triceps, or shoulders or by itself. The same goes for the other muscle groups. Likewise, you shouldn't feel limited to training four consecutive days. Feel free to lift on any four days that work best with your schedule. Table 3.6 shows an example of a four-day split.

TABLE 3.6 Four-Day Split

Day	Muscle groups trained
Monday	Chest, shoulders
Tuesday	Off
Wednesday	Legs
Thursday	Back
Friday	Off
Saturday	Triceps, biceps
Sunday	Off

■ **Five-day split** (frequency of one time per week for each muscle group). Training the entire body over the course of five days allows you to train only one muscle group in most workouts. Many people think this helps them concentrate better on each muscle so that no muscles get short shrift. As with the four-day split, the combinations of muscle pairings and choices of which days to train each muscle group are virtually limitless. Table 3.7 provides an example of a five-day split.

TABLE 3.7 Five-Day Split

Day	Muscle groups trained
Monday	Chest
Tuesday	Back
Wednesday	Legs
Thursday	Off
Friday	Shoulders
Saturday	Triceps, biceps
Sunday	Off

■ **Twice-per-day split** (frequency of one to three times per week for each muscle group). Working out twice a day gives you even more flexibility and allows you to train one muscle group in every workout. This training method is truly for dedicated lifters who have a lifestyle that affords them the luxury of going to the gym twice a day. Training this way gives you the option of working each body part with whatever frequency you like, one to three times a week.

If you choose a twice-per-day split, you'd train one or two muscle groups in each of two daily workouts and would be ready to start over either the next day (for a frequency of three times per week for each muscle group) or two days later (for a frequency of twice per week for each muscle group). Training twice per day, especially if you're doing it six days a week, can easily lead to overtraining. If you choose to do it, you must keep your volume levels in check during each workout (refer to the general volume guidelines in chapter 2 on page 17). In addition, you shouldn't train twice daily for any more than eight weeks. Table 3.8 gives an example of a twice-per-day workout week.

TABLE 3.8   Twice-per-Day Split

Day	Muscle groups trained	
	a.m.	**p.m.**
Monday	Chest	Shoulders, triceps
Tuesday	Legs	Back, biceps
Wednesday	Off	
Thursday	Repeat Monday	
Friday	Repeat Tuesday	
Saturday	Off	
Sunday	Off	

Muscle Matching

As you might have noticed in the sample splits, there are certain consistencies regarding the order in which to train muscle groups. Notice that the biceps and triceps are never trained before the chest, back, or shoulders in the same workout. Always train larger muscles before smaller ones in the same workout. If you were to train your triceps before your chest, your triceps would be tired by the time you started doing pressing exercises for the chest. On such movements, your triceps assist in lifting the weight. If those smaller muscles are fatigued, you won't be able to use as much weight or do as many reps on presses, thereby diminishing the workout your chest muscles get. The same holds true for the back and biceps and even the shoulders and chest. The shoulders are a smaller muscle group than the chest and therefore should be trained after the chest.

Strengths and Weaknesses

A major part of devising an appropriate training split is prioritizing muscle groups based on where your weaknesses lie—weaker muscle groups should generally be given higher priority in order to catch up with your stronger muscles. Giving a muscle group higher priority simply means training it when it's at its strongest, and possibly training it with more volume or frequency. The less fatigued a muscle is, the stronger it will be. For example, the shoulders might be a weak muscle group for you. Since your shoulders are working during most chest exercises, don't work the shoulders after the chest in the same workout. Your shoulders would be fatigued by the time you start devoting your full attention to them. Instead, train the shoulders on a different day than the chest, either alone or with another muscle group that you don't consider a weakness. If your triceps are a strong muscle group, working your shoulders and triceps on the same day (shoulders first, of course) makes sense.

It's also common to find that your chest and back are more developed than your arms. If this is the case, the simple solution to developing your arms is to not train the triceps on the same day as the chest or the biceps with the back, as many people do. Instead, devote one workout entirely to your arms, and make sure they're not still fatigued from a chest or back workout you did the day before. Tables 3.9 through 3.12 provide examples of splits designed around weaknesses in various muscle groups.

TABLE 3.9   Weakness: Shoulders (Four-Day Split)

Day	Muscle groups trained
Monday	Chest, triceps
Tuesday	Back, biceps, forearms
Wednesday	Legs
Thursday	Off
Friday	Shoulders
Saturday	Off
Sunday	Off

TABLE 3.10   Weakness: Arms (Five-Day Split)

Day	Muscle groups trained
Monday	Triceps, biceps
Tuesday	Legs
Wednesday	Chest, back
Thursday	Off
Friday	Triceps, biceps
Saturday	Shoulders
Sunday	Off

TABLE 3.11 **Weakness: Chest (Four-Day Split)**

Day	Muscle groups trained
Monday	Chest
Tuesday	Back, biceps
Wednesday	Legs, shoulders
Thursday	Off
Friday	Chest, triceps
Saturday	Off
Sunday	Off

TABLE 3.12 **Weakness: Back (Four-Day Split)**

Day	Muscle groups trained
Monday	Back
Tuesday	Chest, shoulders
Wednesday	Legs
Thursday	Off
Friday	Back, biceps
Saturday	Off
Sunday	Off

Different Muscles and Different Frequencies

Not every muscle group has to be trained with the same frequency. Just because you train your chest and back twice a week doesn't mean you have to do your shoulders twice a week too. Notice in tables 3.9 through 3.12 how the weak body part in each split not only is given priority within its workout (or given its own workout altogether) but is also given ample rest before the day it's trained. For example, your shoulders might still be fatigued the day after training your chest, but they should be well rested if you trained your legs the day before. Also notice that in some examples the weak muscle group is trained more frequently than strong ones. The point is to train the lagging areas with higher volume over the course of the week.

Split Extensions

Just as splits don't always need to be symmetrical in terms of muscle frequency, your split does not have to be based on a seven-day cycle. To this point we've only discussed splits in terms of one-week spans, after which you would start over the next week. But we do this only for simplicity's sake. If you want to train each muscle group with a frequency of twice per week but can't quite fit it into seven days, extend your split to 8 to 10 days, then start over from there. The major difference is that your split will begin on a different day every week, which shouldn't be a problem, especially if you keep a training log.

Extending the split past seven days works well for those who want to train each muscle group once a week in some weeks and twice a week in others. Take, for example, a three-day split in which you want to rest two days after working the whole body so that you're doing a continual three-days-on, two-days-off regimen. In this case, you'll train the entire body once every 5 days (including off days) and twice every 10 days. The result is a split, such as that shown in table 3.13, in which every muscle is trained either once or twice per week.

TABLE 3.13   Sample 10-Day Split

Day	Muscle groups trained
Monday	Back, shoulders
Tuesday	Legs
Wednesday	Chest, triceps, biceps
Thursday	Off
Friday	Off
Saturday	Back, shoulders
Sunday	Legs
Monday	Chest, triceps
Tuesday	Off
Wednesday	Off
Cycle repeats.	

Split Variations

Your training split doesn't have to be the same every week. Even if you decide to stick to a four-day split for a time, those four days can be different from week to week. Consider a basic four-day split in which you'd like to change the emphasis every week from the chest to the back to the shoulders so that each week one of those three muscle groups receives the undivided attention of its own workout. Simply rotate the muscles you train on days 1 and 2 of each week, keeping days 3 and 4 constant (legs on day 3, arms on day 4). Table 3.14 shows how you could vary your split over the course of three weeks.

TABLE 3.14   Three-Week Alternating Split

Week 1	Week 2	Week 3
Day 1: Chest	Back	Shoulders
Day 2: Back, shoulders	Chest, shoulders	Chest, back
Days 3 and 4 are legs and arms, respectively.		

TYPES OF LIFTING EXERCISES

It's assumed that you wouldn't do just one exercise per muscle group (unless you're training with a three-times-per-week frequency with only 3 or 4 sets per muscle group in each workout). If you're doing 12 to 15 sets for a given muscle group in a workout, you would split those sets into three to five different exercises and do 3 to 5 sets each. Using different exercises with different angles and varying movements allows you to completely develop the muscles involved. The chapters that follow describe specific exercises; however, all lifting exercises fall into at least one of the following categories.

Free-Weight Exercises (Barbells, Dumbbells)

If you're serious about lifting, regardless of your goal, the foundation of your program should be free-weight exercises. Exercises performed with barbells and dumbbells allow a free range of motion and require the use of more stabilizing muscle groups, which are required for gaining more strength and preventing injury. And when using free weights, you can be sure that resistance is supported and lifted solely by you, not by a machine dictating the path of motion.

You'll find that you're able to lift more total weight on barbell movements than when using dumbbells. If you can do 10 reps with 70-pound dumbbells on the flat bench press, chances are you can do significantly more reps with 140 pounds (70 pounds times 2) on the barbell bench press. Because each dumbbell must be balanced individually (isolaterally), your muscles are required to do more work to keep the weights steady, thus decreasing their capacity to simply press the dumbbells up. One advantage of using dumbbells over a barbell is that a stronger limb can't compensate for a weaker arm or leg, promoting balance in both sides of the body.

Machine Exercises (Cambered Machines, Cables, Smith Machine)

Although free-weight exercises should take priority in your training, machines are crucial too. Machines are typically safer and almost never require a spotter. Moreover, because you tend not to use as many stabilizing muscles when doing a machine lift, you'll be able to overload the target muscle with more weight. For example, on a chest press machine, the path is already set for you, allowing you to rely less on stabilizing muscles that might tire out before the target muscles, in this case the pectorals.

Cable equipment is unique in that it allows force to be applied to a muscle in a variety of directions, whereas free-weight exercises must be performed only vertically to work against gravity. Cables also provide tension on the muscles through the entire range of motion, an added benefit over some free-weight exercises. With barbell or dumbbell preacher curls, for example, the tension is not squarely on the biceps at the top of the motion when the bar is directly over your elbows; rather, the bar is being supported by the bones of the forearms at this point. Constant tension would be better achieved by doing *cable* preacher curls instead of barbell or dumbbell preacher curls.

Cam-based machines, like cables, allow for movements in various directions with constant tension. But they also mimic the strength curve of the muscle so that the perception of resistance is the same throughout the entire range of motion, instead of varying at different points along the path of motion as with free-weight exercises.

In addition to the technical benefits, machines add variety to your routine. Weight machines are becoming more innovative and effective and can make up an effective program by themselves if necessary. In fact, some muscle groups, such as the back, lend themselves better to machines. Without machine exercises, you'd be limited to pull-ups and free-weight rows, and you'd miss out on lat pull-downs and cable rows, which are mainstays in most elite bodybuilders' and athletes' back workouts.

Unilateral and Bilateral Movements

Virtually any movement can be done either with one arm (unilaterally) or with two arms (bilaterally) at a time. Unilateral exercises typically require using either a dumbbell or a cable handle, although you can do most machine exercises one arm at a time if you lighten the weight accordingly. A normal dumbbell press, for instance, is done two arms at a time, despite the fact that each arm works independently. To focus even more on each arm, do the press using only one arm; you can hold on to the bench with the other arm to steady yourself. Unilateral training is helpful if you have a weak arm or leg that you want to make as strong as the other one, and it's an easy way to add variety to your workout. Research shows that unilateral training allows you to lift more weight with the one arm than that arm would lift doing the exercise bilaterally, and it enhances core strength as well.

Compound and Isolation Exercises

A compound exercise is one in which multiple joints are involved. One of many examples is a rowing exercise for back, in which both shoulder and elbow joints are initiating the movement; other examples are chest and shoulder presses. Isolation exercises involve movement at only one joint. Examples are biceps curls and triceps extensions, in which only the elbow moves; lateral raises for the shoulders, in which the elbows remain stationary and only the shoulders are working; and flys for the chest, where again, only the shoulder joints move.

Because they involve multiple joints and call on more muscles to help move the weight, compound exercises are better for building size and strength because you're able to lift more weight. For smaller muscle groups such as biceps and triceps, most exercises involve only one joint (the elbow in this case). You can train triceps by doing close-grip bench presses and dips, both compound movements, but you'll find that virtually every other triceps exercise is a single-joint move.

EXERCISE ORDER

Just as your training split requires mindful organization in order to be effective, you must carefully plan the order in which you do exercises. Though there are exceptions to nearly every rule, some general guidelines can help you determine the best order of exercises.

One guideline is to perform compound exercises before isolation exercises of the same muscle group. Generally speaking, you should do exercises that allow you to lift the most weight (compound exercises) early in your workout. For example, if you plan to do two pressing movements for chest and one fly movement, do your flys after presses. (One exception to this rule is a technique known as preexhaustion, which is discussed in chapter 10.)

You should also perform free-weight exercises before machine exercises. So, if you plan to do two pressing exercises (a barbell press and a machine press), do the barbell press first. If the machine exercise happens to be a compound exercise and the free-weight exercise is an isolation exercise, follow the previous guideline and perform the compound exercise first. But, again, this isn't a hard-and-fast rule—many advanced lifters flip-flop the order on occasion with good results.

Another guideline is that barbell exercises should be performed before dumbbell exercises. An example is doing a barbell incline press before a dumbbell flat bench press. You will likely be able to lift more weight on the barbell exercise, so to maximize gains in size and strength, do the barbell exercise when your muscles are fresh; that way you'll be able to use more weight. If you are planning on doing two barbell pressing movements, such as incline and flat bench, you could do either first.

Finally, you should prioritize your exercises based on weaknesses. For the previous example, when deciding whether to do the flat bench or incline press first, keep in mind where your weaknesses lie. If your upper pectorals are underdeveloped in relation to your middle and lower pectorals, do the inclines, which emphasize the upper pectorals, first.

REP RANGES AND RESISTANCE

The number of reps you should do in a given set depends on your training goal. Furthermore, the weight you choose to lift on a given set depends on the number of reps you're going for, which is why the two variables—reps and resistance—go hand in hand. As noted in chapter 2, select a weight that will cause you to reach failure on the last set or two of the exercise. As for the number of reps to do, here's what we recommend based on individual goals:

■ **Muscular strength.** When strength is the primary goal, the optimal rep range per set is three to six. The objective is to overload your muscles with as much weight as they can handle over a very short period, which won't allow for a lot of reps. Strength is defined as the maximum amount of weight you can lift one time and is typically measured by low-rep maximum lifts, such as a one-rep, three-rep, or five-rep max. Conditioning your muscles to handle maximal loads is the key to developing all-out strength.

■ **Muscular size.** Your muscles will grow when you train for strength, but not as much as they will when you do slightly more reps per set. Hence, the optimal rep range for maximal size is 8 to 12. In this range, combine relatively heavy weight with a sufficient number of reps to increase the muscles' time under tension, or the amount of time a muscle contracts in a single bout, which causes the muscle fibers to grow.

If you want a combination of strength and size, your reps should fall in the top end of the strength range and the low end of the hypertrophy range, somewhere around six to eight. It's very common for serious lifters to consistently do sets of eight reps to reap the benefits of both strength and hypertrophy training.

■ **Muscular endurance.** Increasing the endurance of your muscles is often confused with achieving more muscular definition. Often you'll hear people say that doing higher reps (15 to 20 or more) helps you get more defined than lower rep ranges. It's not quite that simple. Increasing definition requires losing body fat, which is achieved through healthful eating habits as well as exercise. Working in the 8- to 12-rep range is as effective for developing muscular definition, if not more effective, than doing sets of 15, 20, or more. Doing sets of 15 or more reps is ideal for increasing muscular endurance, which is especially helpful if you compete in endurance sports such as cross country running, cycling, and swimming.

Just as you don't have to train every muscle group with the same frequency, nor must you follow the same rep ranges for your entire body. You might want to train your chest, back, and shoulders for strength with low reps but train your arms with 8 to 12 reps to add size to them. And some muscle groups simply respond better to high reps than to low reps. You might find that your back responds better to high reps than your chest does. If this is the case, train the two groups differently. Trial and error is the best way to find out what works for you.

Regardless of your goal, it's essential to alter your rep ranges from time to time. If you train your arms with 10-rep sets week after week, they will get accustomed to that rep range and will stagnate. You need to train them on occasion with lower reps (6 per set) and higher reps (15 per set). Even though these rep ranges are best suited for strength and endurance, respectively, combining them with a rep range that promotes hypertrophy is the best way to make continued gains. The same holds true when training for strength. There are numerous ways to go about changing or cycling your rep ranges, known formally as periodization, which are illustrated in the training programs in chapter 11.

Rest Periods

How long to rest between sets typically corresponds to the particular rep range you're working in (see table 3.15). If you're training for strength in the three- to six-rep range, rest longer between sets (around two to five minutes). To gain strength, ensure that your muscles are as close to fully rested as possible for each set. Don't risk less-than-full recovery with shorter rest periods simply to speed up your workout.

TABLE 3.15 **The Three Rs: Reps, Resistance, Rest**

Goal	Rep range and resistance	Rest periods between sets
Strength	3-6 reps/heavy	2-5 minutes
Size (hypertrophy)	8-12 reps/moderate to heavy	60-90 seconds
Endurance	15-30 reps/light to moderate	20-45 seconds

On the other end of the spectrum, developing endurance requires continuous, or at least near-continuous, bouts of exercise. So if you're training for endurance with high reps, short rest periods of around 30 seconds are ideal. Resting for longer than you're working defeats the whole purpose.

If you're doing reps of 8 to 12 for hypertrophy, anywhere from 60 to 90 seconds is optimal. Hypertrophy training falls somewhere in the middle—you don't want your muscles to be fully rested between sets (as with strength training), but rest periods that are too brief will decrease the number of reps you're able to do on subsequent sets.

Rep Speed

Every repetition you do in the gym is composed of a concentric, or positive, phase (also referred to as the exertion phase) and an eccentric, or negative, phase (in which you resist or lower the weight between concentric phases). On a bench press, overhead press, or biceps curl, the concentric is the "up" phase and the eccentric is the "down" portion of the rep; on a lat pull-down, however, it's just the opposite—the concentric is when you pull down, the eccentric is when you let the bar up. And while the concentric portion may seem to be the more important of the two, both portions are equally important in developing muscular size, strength, and endurance. In fact, the soreness you feel in your muscles the day after a hard lifting session is caused more by the negative phase of reps than the positive.

How fast you should complete each rep varies depending on your goal, but generally speaking, the concentric phase should be around one to three seconds in duration, and the eccentric phase should be around two to four seconds. The time depends on how much weight you're using and how fatigued you are—if the weight is extremely heavy, or if you're at the very end of a demanding set to failure, you may find it takes you a few seconds to lift the weight, whereas with a lighter weight under less fatigue the concentric phase is much quicker. However, don't feel you need to count the seconds it takes you to lift or lower a weight; on the negative, for instance, the important thing is that you lower the weight under control (as opposed to simply letting it drop), whether that means four seconds or a second and a half.

Breathing

How to breathe during the course of each rep is a somewhat debated topic. You've likely been told before that you should inhale on the eccentric portion of the rep and exhale on the concentric. But for maximizing your strength on each rep, this advice is only partially correct. The problem is that when someone tells you to exhale on the concentric, that person usually means exhale the entire way up. A more effective way is to inhale on the eccentric, hold your breath through most of the concentric, then exhale completely as you're finishing the rep. This may sound unorthodox, even dangerous, but if you're healthy it's safe and will allow you to perform more reps per set. If you have any preexisting heart condition, high blood pressure, or other physical ailment, however, consult a physician before doing any intense weight training.

WARM-UPS AND FLEXIBILITY

Preparing your body for intense training is a vital practice at the beginning of every lifting session. The warm-up, however, shouldn't take very long, because you don't want to tire yourself out before the workout begins. Begin with light cardiorespiratory exercise for 5 to 10 minutes, which you can do on any piece of equipment you find at the gym, such as a treadmill, stair stepper, or stationary bike. The pace should be low to moderate in intensity, just enough to raise your body temperature above its normal state.

After that, you can begin lifting, but always with warm-up sets before going heavy. On the first exercise for each muscle group, do at least one set of that exercise with a light weight (never to failure) before doing your first working set. For example, if the bench press is your first exercise on a day when you're working your chest and triceps and you plan to lift 200 pounds for 10 reps for your first working set, do a set of 10 reps with 135 pounds first, and then 5 to 8 reps with 185 pounds before jumping up to 200. After doing your working sets on the bench, you'll likely find you don't need any warm-up sets on the chest exercises that follow. You should, however, do a warm-up set or two on your first triceps exercise.

When, how, and how much to stretch is an often-misunderstood topic. Avoid stretching before your muscles are warmed up, which can lead to muscle strains and pulls. Many athletes will do a light cardiorespiratory warm-up before stretching to avoid such injuries, then begin the workout. Technically, there's nothing wrong with this; but where lifting is concerned, stretching before training has been shown in numerous scientific studies to decrease strength in the ensuing workout. Therefore, you should not stretch (just warm up) before lifting, assuming it's important to you that you be as strong as possible during your workout.

Even if your goal is to improve muscular endurance, you should still use as heavy a weight as possible for high reps. But this does not mean you shouldn't stretch. Flexibility is important for avoiding muscular injuries and enhancing overall physical performance. Do your stretching after you lift, when strength levels won't be affected and your muscles will be warmed up from the preceding workout. Stretching only the muscles you just trained should suffice, unless you have more ambitious flexibility goals. In that case, you can stretch other muscles, provided they're sufficiently warmed up.

PART II

Upper-Body Exercises

CHAPTER 4

Chest Exercises

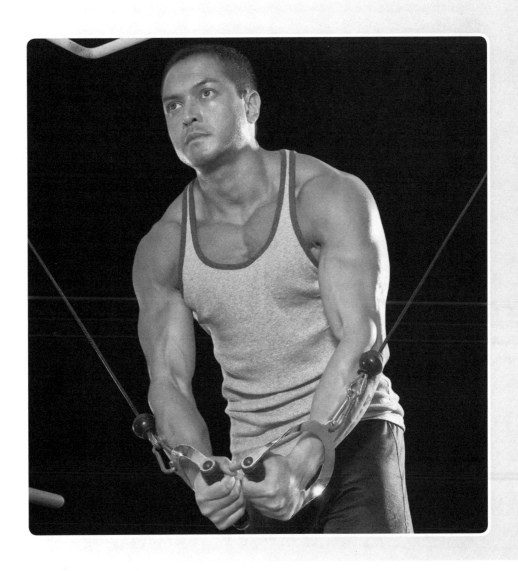

Chest exercises can be broken down into two major types: presses and flys. Presses include all barbell, dumbbell, and machine presses performed on a flat, incline, or decline bench and are considered compound movements because both the shoulder and elbow joints are initiating the movement (dips are also considered a pressing exercise). Flys, which can be done with dumbbells, using cables (sometimes called crossovers), or on a machine, isolate the pectoral muscles with minimal involvement from the triceps. As noted in chapter 3, presses should typically be done before flys in a chest workout (unless using the preexhaustion technique, which is explained in chapter 10). In addition to presses and flys, a third and somewhat less major chest movement is the pull-over, another isolation motion to be done later in a workout.

Which pressing exercise to perform first (flat, incline, or decline) depends on which area of the pectorals you want to focus on. If your upper pectorals are weak in relation to your middle and lower pectorals, do incline presses first. If you have no significant weakness in any one area of the chest, vary which press you do first—alternate between flat bench and incline presses every other workout (flat bench presses also involve the lower pectorals, so the decline is rarely suggested as a first exercise). The same advice applies to fly movements. If your upper pectorals are a weakness, focus on incline flys rather than flat bench or decline flys.

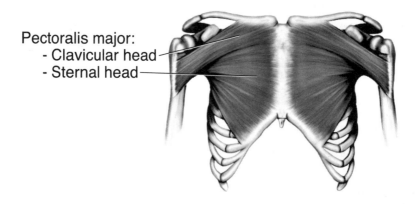

Pectoralis major:
- Clavicular head
- Sternal head

BARBELL BENCH PRESS

Target	Middle pectorals
When	Early in workout
Start	Lie back on a flat bench with a rack. Grasp the bar with your hands just outside shoulder width, unrack the bar, and begin with it directly over your upper pectorals with your arms extended.
Execution	Bend your elbows to slowly lower the bar toward your lower chest. Touch your chest lightly with the bar, then press it back up in a slight backward arcing motion so the bar ends up over your upper chest with your arms extended but not locked out.
Variations	Take a wider grip to target the outer pectorals. Take a narrower grip (but no closer than shoulder width; otherwise the triceps are targeted) for the inner pectorals.
Advanced Tip	Place your feet together up on the end of the bench or up in the air, which requires extra balance and calls on more core and stabilizing muscles.
Substitutes	Dumbbell press—flat bench, Smith machine bench press, Hammer Strength chest press, machine press

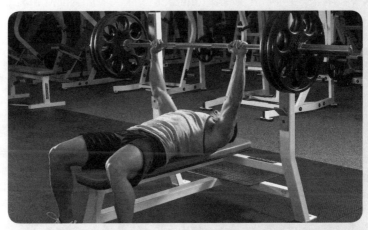

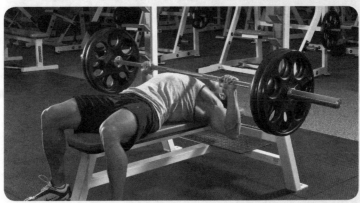

SMITH MACHINE BENCH PRESS

Target	Middle pectorals
When	Early in workout
Start	Position a flat bench in a Smith machine and position it so the bar touches your lower chest at the bottom of each rep. Make sure the bench is centered in the machine so as not to favor either side. Lie back on the bench, grasp the bar outside shoulder width, unhook the latches, and begin with your arms extended.
Execution	Slowly lower the bar down to your chest, touch down lightly, then press the bar back up to the arms-extended position without locking out your elbows. After the desired number of reps, rerack the bar.
Variations	Use an incline or a decline bench to target either the upper or lower pectorals. For the incline, lower the bar to your upper chest; for the decline, touch down to your lower pectorals.
Advanced Tip	Set the safety guards so that the bar doesn't quite reach your chest at the bottom, and begin each set in the down position. On each rep, rest the bar on the guards for a split second at the bottom; this will eliminate momentum from the eccentric portion.
Substitutes	Barbell bench press, dumbbell press—flat bench, machine press

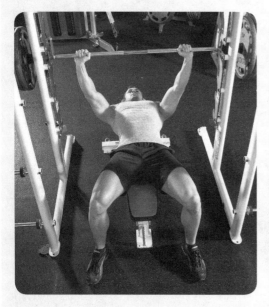 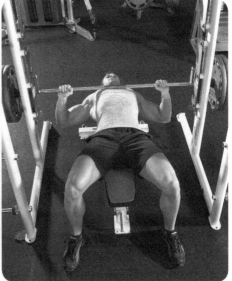

MACHINE PRESS

Target
Middle pectorals

When
After barbell or dumbbell presses but before fly movements

Start
Adjust the seat of a machine press so that the handles are outside your lower chest in the down position. Keep your feet flat on the floor and your back and head against the seat back. Begin in the down position.

Execution
Press the weight along the predetermined path of motion until your elbows are extended but not locked out. Slowly lower the bar to the down position without letting the weight rest on the stack between reps.

Variations
There are many types of machine presses, including ones that mimic decline and incline presses and plate-loaded machines (Hammer Strength, pictured, is one of the more popular brands). Many also have various grip positions, which allows you to use a very wide or narrower grip and even a neutral grip.

Advanced Tip
Machines that use a weight stack provide a convenient means of doing drop sets (see page 186 in chapter 10); decreasing the weight after reaching failure is as simple as moving the pin up.

Substitutes
Barbell bench press, dumbbell press—flat bench, Smith machine bench press

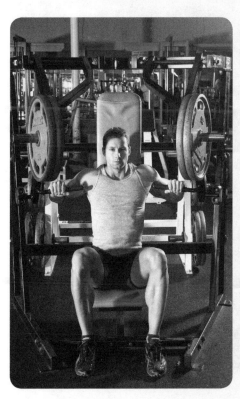 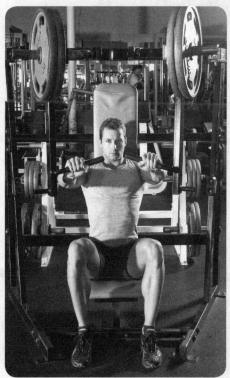

PUSH-UP

Target	Middle pectorals
When	To warm up, near the end of the workout, or when you have no other equipment
Start	Place your hands about shoulder-width apart flat on the floor, with your body flat and rigid and your toes on the floor. Begin with your arms extended, perpendicular to the floor.
Execution	Bend your elbows to slowly lower yourself down to the floor. When your chest reaches a few inches from touching, extend your elbows to forcefully press yourself back up to the start position.
Variations	To emphasize the upper chest and increase difficulty, place your feet up on a bench, chair, or couch (depending on where you are) for the entire set. To emphasize the lower chest and decrease difficulty, place your hands on an elevated, stable surface.
Advanced Tip	Instead of having your hands on the floor, place them on an exercise ball or medicine ball (keep your feet on the floor behind you). This will require a high level of balance and will train the stabilizing muscles and the core.
Substitutes	Barbell bench press, dumbbell press—flat bench, Smith machine press, machine press (use a light weight with all)

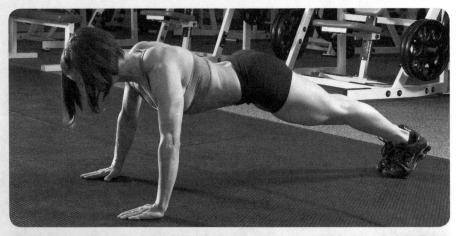

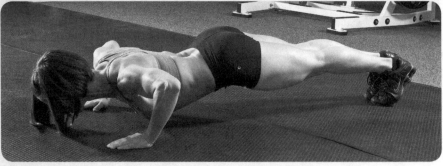

DUMBBELL PRESS—FLAT BENCH

Target	Middle pectorals
When	Early in workout
Start	Lie faceup on a flat bench while holding a pair of dumbbells just outside your chest with your elbows bent and palms facing forward.
Execution	Contract your pectorals and extend your arms to press the dumbbells straight up and together over your chest, keeping your palms facing forward. Don't lock out your elbows at the top. Slowly lower the dumbbells back to the start position.
Variations	As you press the dumbbells up, turn your palms in to face each other at the top of each rep and squeeze your pectorals together for a more intense contraction. Or perform dumbbell presses using a neutral grip (palms facing each other) throughout the entire range of motion to involve more of the upper pectorals.
Advanced Tip	Perform this exercise one arm at a time, using your nonworking hand to hold on to the bench below your leg for stability. This will likely require using a lighter dumbbell.
Substitutes	Barbell bench press, Smith machine press, Hammer Strength chest press, machine press

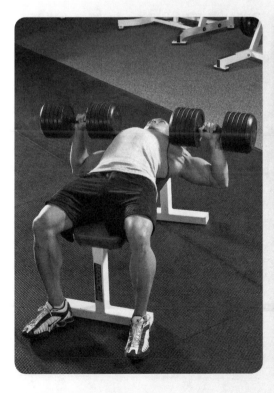 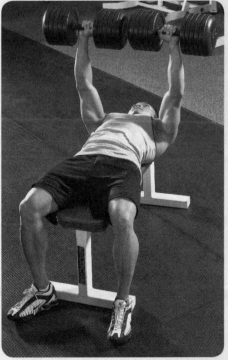

DUMBBELL FLY–FLAT BENCH

Target	Middle and outer pectorals
When	Late in workout
Start	Lie back on a flat bench while holding a pair of dumbbells. Begin with the weights held together and directly over you, palms in, with your elbows slightly bent.
Execution	Maintaining only a slight bend in your elbows, slowly lower the dumbbells in a wide arc out to either side until you feel a stretch in your chest. Contract your pectorals to return the weights to the start position, keeping your elbows fixed in the slightly bent position throughout. Squeeze your pectorals together at the top.
Variation	As you lift the weights up, turn your palms inward (supination) so that by the top of each rep your forearms face you. Squeeze your pectorals hard in this position.
Advanced Tip	To keep constant tension on your pectorals, stop about 12 inches shy of the dumbbells' touching each other at the top of each rep.
Substitutes	Machine fly, cable crossover, cable fly

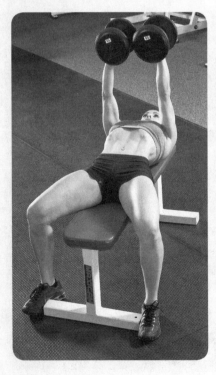 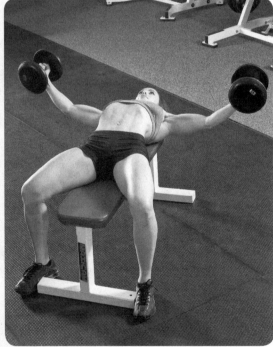

CABLE FLY

Target	Middle, inner, and outer pectorals
When	Late in workout
Start	Position a flat bench equidistant between two cable stacks and adjust both pulleys, with handles attached, to low settings on their respective columns. Grab hold of the handles and lie back on the bench. Your shoulders should be roughly in line with the pulleys. Begin with your arms slightly bent and out to your sides with your hands at chest level.
Execution	Maintaining the slight bend in your elbows, contract your pectorals to pull your hands together in an arcing motion over your chest. When your hands reach each other, squeeze your pectorals hard for a count for full contraction. Slowly return to the start position.
Variations	Perform the cable fly with an incline or decline bench to target the upper or lower pectorals, respectively. On the incline, pull the handles up over your upper chest; on the decline, pull them over your lower chest.
Advanced Tip	At the top of each rep, cross your hands over one another so that your wrists touch. Squeeze your pectorals together in this position.
Substitutes	Cable crossover, machine fly, dumbbell fly—flat bench

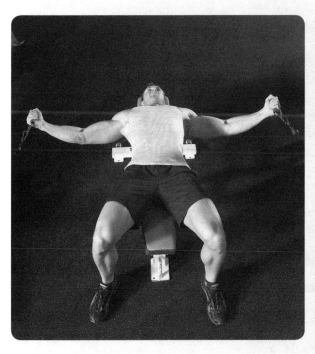
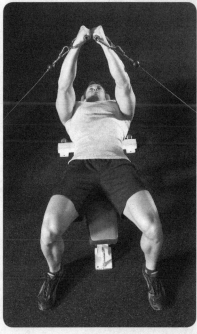

MACHINE FLY

Target   Outer and inner pectorals

When   End of workout

Start   Adjust the seat of a fly machine so that the handles are at chest level. Sit on the seat with your back flat against the pad, grasp the handles, and begin with your arms straight out to the sides and your elbows slightly bent.

Execution   Contract your pectorals to bring your hands together. When your hands touch, squeeze your pectorals hard for a count, then slowly return to the start position without letting the weight rest on the stack.

Variation   Some fly machines (sometimes referred to as pec decks) include arm pads to place the insides of your elbows and forearms on while keeping your elbows bent at roughly a 90-degree angle throughout the motion.

Advanced Tip   Adjust the seat up or down to target different areas of the chest. Sitting higher up emphasizes the lower pectorals; sitting lower emphasizes the upper pectorals.

Substitutes   Cable crossover, cable fly, dumbbell fly—flat bench

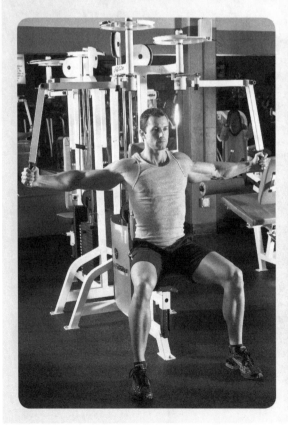
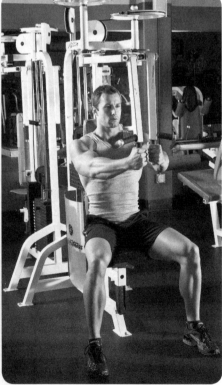

EXERCISE BALL DUMBBELL PRESS—ADVANCED

Target   Middle chest, core, and stabilizing muscles

When   Early in workout

Start   While holding two relatively light dumbbells, place your back on an exercise ball. Look up toward the ceiling; bend your knees and place your feet apart and flat on the floor. Begin with your elbows bent and the dumbbells just outside your chest, with your palms facing forward.

Execution   While concentrating on maintaining your balance on the ball, press the dumbbells straight up over your chest until your arms are extended but not locked out. Carefully lower the dumbbells back to the start position.

Variation   To emphasize the upper pectorals, lower your hips so that your torso is approximately 45 degrees to the floor (your buttocks will be almost touching the floor in this position) and press the weight straight up.

Advanced Tip   As you press the dumbbells up, turn your wrists inward so that your forearms face each other at the top of each rep.

Substitutes   Dumbbell press—flat bench, push-up

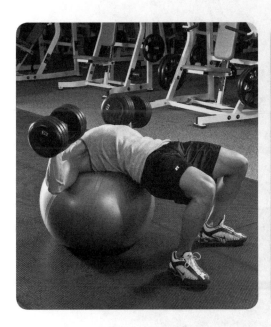 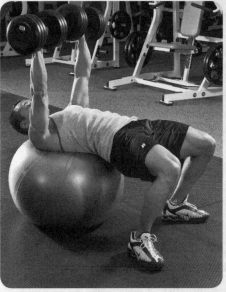

EXERCISE BALL DUMBBELL FLY—ADVANCED

Target   Middle and outer pectorals, core, and stabilizing muscles

When   End of workout

Start   While holding two light dumbbells, place your back on an exercise ball. Look up toward the ceiling; bend your knees, and place your feet apart and flat on the floor. Begin with the dumbbells over your chest, with your elbows slightly bent and your palms facing each other.

Execution   Maintaining only a slight bend in your elbows, slowly lower the dumbbells in an arc out to the sides until you feel a stretch in your chest. Contract your pectorals to return the dumbbells to the start position.

Variation   Target the upper pectorals by lowering your hips so that your torso is approximately 45 degrees with the floor.

Advanced Tip   To increase difficulty, perform the exercise with only one foot on the floor and the other suspended in the air or resting on the opposite knee.

Substitutes   Dumbbell fly—flat bench, cable fly, machine fly, cable crossover

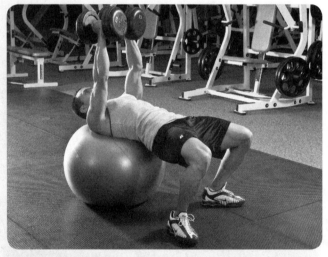

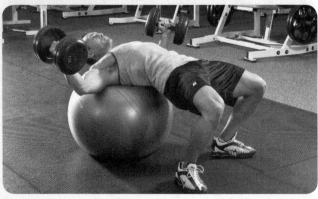

ASSISTED DIP–MACHINE

Target
Middle and lower pectorals

When
After pressing exercises but before fly movements

Start
Select a weight that will assist you in reaching failure at your desired number of reps. Begin by holding on to the bars, with your body vertical to the floor, your arms extended, and your feet on the pegs.

Execution
Bend your arms to slowly lower yourself down while simultaneously leaning slightly forward with your upper body. When your elbows reach roughly 90 degrees, press yourself back up to the start position.

Variation
A similar exercise involves a seated dip machine, which many gyms have. Be sure to lean forward (instead of sitting back against the pad) to emphasize the pectorals, not the triceps.

Advanced Tip
Begin the set with a light weight (which makes it more difficult), go to failure, then set the pin to a heavier weight (making it easier) and go to failure. Repeat for one or two more drop sets.

Substitutes
Dip—wide grip, decline barbell press, decline dumbbell press

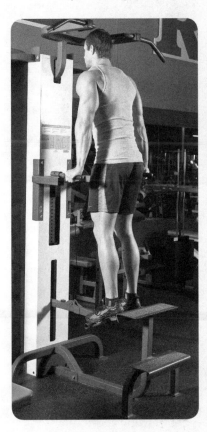 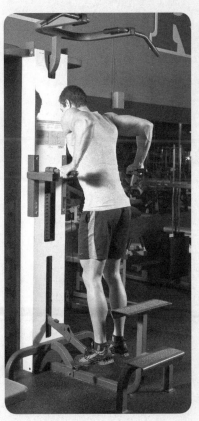

DIP—WIDE GRIP

Target   Middle and lower pectorals

When   After pressing exercises but before fly movements

Start   Find a dip apparatus with relatively wide grips (at least shoulder width). Begin by holding on to the bars, with your body vertical to the floor and your arms extended.

Execution   Bend your arms to slowly lower yourself down while simultaneously leaning slightly forward with your upper body. When your elbows reach roughly 90 degrees, press yourself back up to the start position.

Variation   Keeping your body upright (not leaning forward) deemphasizes the pectorals and trains the triceps to a greater extent (see dip—narrow grip on page 131).

Advanced Tip   Perform dips with extra weight (weighted dips) by hanging a weight plate or dumbbell from a chain attached to a lifting belt.

Substitutes   Assisted dip—machine, decline barbell press, decline dumbbell press

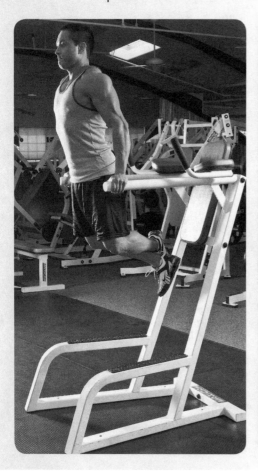 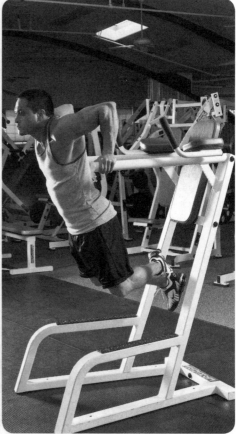

DUMBBELL PULL-OVER

Target   Middle and lower pectorals

When   Late in workout

Start   Lie with your shoulder blades resting on a flat bench and your body extended out perpendicular to the bench, feet flat on the floor and knees bent. Hold one dumbbell with both hands. Drop your hips below the level of the bench, and begin by holding the dumbbell straight up over your chest with your arms straight.

Execution   With your elbows slightly bent, lower the dumbbell back and behind your head until you feel a stretch in your pectorals and upper arms. Contract your pectorals to return the dumbbell to the start position, maintaining only a slight bend in your elbows.

Variations   Perform pull-overs using a barbell with the same technique or on a specialized pull-over machine.

Advanced Tip   To involve more stabilizing muscles, use two light dumbbells (one in each hand) instead of one heavier dumbbell. Keep your wrists in a neutral position (palms facing each other) throughout. After reaching failure, continue the set by doing neutral-grip dumbbell presses (superset, preexhaustion; see pages 182 and 194).

Substitutes   Barbell pull-over, machine pull-over

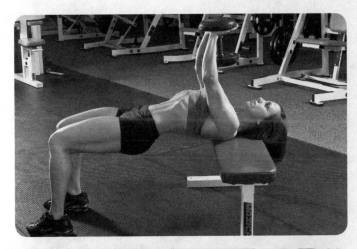

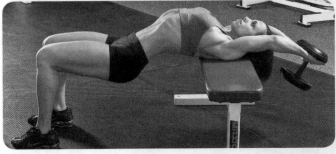

INCLINE BARBELL PRESS

Target   Upper pectorals

When   Early in workout

Start   Lie back on an incline bench (set to 45 degrees) with a rack and grasp the bar with an overhand grip outside of shoulder width. Unrack the bar, and start with it directly over your upper chest, arms extended.

Execution   Slowly lower the bar to your upper chest by bending your elbows. Touch the bar to your chest lightly, then press it back up to the start position without locking out your elbows.

Variation   If you have shoulder problems, stop short of touching your chest at the bottom of each rep.

Advanced Tip   Instead of going immediately up with the bar after lowering it, pause for a count at the bottom of each rep before pressing the weight up. This eliminates all momentum and elastic recoil.

Substitutes   Incline dumbbell press, Smith machine incline press, Hammer Strength incline press, machine incline press

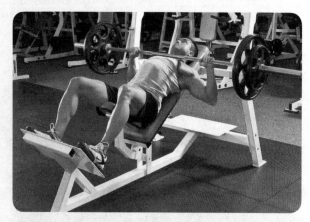

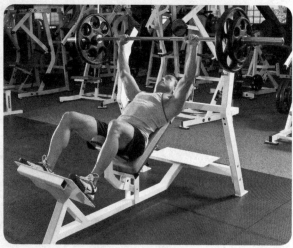

INCLINE DUMBBELL PRESS

Target	Upper pectorals
When	Early in workout
Start	Lie back on an adjustable incline bench set to a 45-degree angle. Hold a pair of dumbbells just outside your shoulders with your palms facing forward.
Execution	Press the dumbbells straight up by contracting your pectorals and extending your arms until your elbows are just short of locked out. Slowly lower the dumbbells back to the start position.
Variation	To work more of the middle chest while still emphasizing the upper pectorals, perform incline presses at less than a 45-degree angle.
Advanced Tip	To work the pectorals at a slightly different angle, perform this exercise with your palms facing in (neutral) throughout the set. For variety, alternate palms forward and palms neutral every other set.
Substitutes	Incline barbell press, Smith machine incline press, Hammer Strength upper chest press, incline machine press

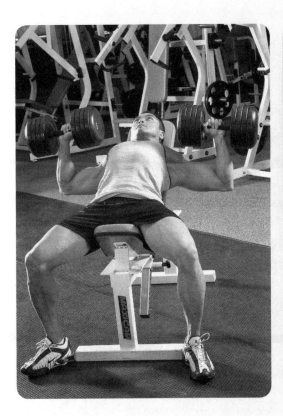
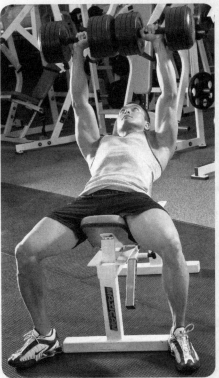

INCLINE DUMBBELL FLY

Target   Upper and outer pectorals

When   Late in workout

Start   Lie back on an incline bench set to approximately a 45-degree angle while holding a pair of dumbbells. Begin with the weights held together over your face with your palms in and your elbows slightly bent.

Execution   Maintaining the slight bend in your elbows, lower the weights down and out to the sides until you feel a stretch in your chest. Contract your pectorals to return the dumbbells to the start position, squeezing the contraction at the top.

Variation   As with the flat bench fly, try turning your palms toward you as you lift the dumbbells, then squeeze your pectorals at the top.

Advanced Tip   After reaching failure, continue the set by going directly into incline dumbbell presses until reaching failure again (superset; see page 182).

Substitutes   Low pulley cable crossover, incline cable fly

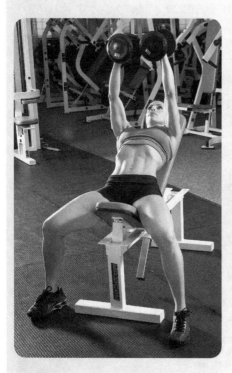 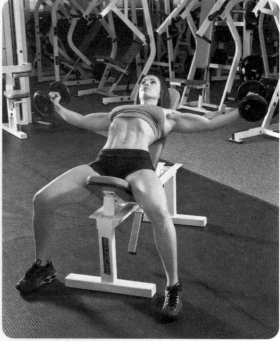

DECLINE BARBELL PRESS

Target	Lower pectorals
When	After flat or incline presses but before fly movements
Start	Lie back on a decline bench with a rack. Secure your feet underneath the ankle pads. Grasp the bar at slightly wider than shoulder width and unrack it. Start with the bar directly over your lower chest and your arms extended.
Execution	Bend your elbows to slowly lower the bar to your lower pectorals, touch it lightly to your chest, then press the bar straight up to the start position without locking out your elbows at the top.
Variation	To hit more of the middle chest, adjust the bench (if possible) to only a slight decline. Decline presses don't need to be performed at a steep angle.
Advanced Tip	For a stronger contraction, squeeze your pectorals together at the top of each rep, as if you're trying to bend the bar.
Substitutes	Decline dumbbell press, Hammer Strength decline press, Smith machine decline press, dip—wide grip

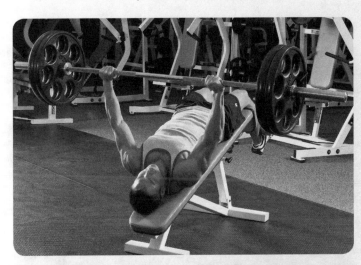

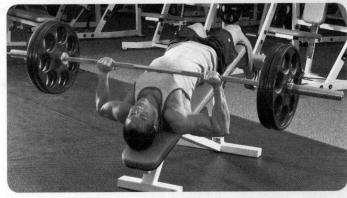

DECLINE DUMBBELL PRESS

Target	Lower pectorals
When	After flat or incline presses but before fly movements
Start	Lie back on a decline bench while holding a pair of dumbbells just outside your lower chest with your elbows bent and feet secured underneath the ankle pads and palms facing forward.
Execution	Press the dumbbells straight up over your chest by contracting your pectorals and extending your arms until your elbows are just short of locked out. Slowly lower the dumbbells down to the start position.
Variation	If a steep decline is uncomfortable in any way, adjust the bench to only a slight decline, which will still emphasize the lower pectorals.
Advanced Tip	As you press the weights up, turn your wrists toward each other so that at the top of the rep your forearms face in and the dumbbells touch. Squeeze your pectorals hard in this position.
Substitutes	Decline barbell press, Smith machine decline press, Hammer Strength decline press, dip—wide grip

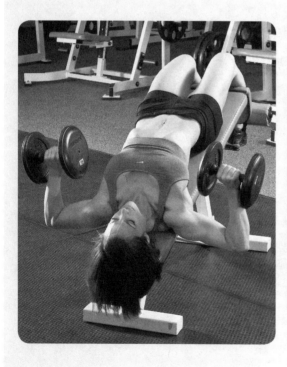 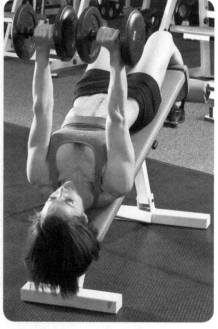

DECLINE DUMBBELL FLY

Target	Lower and outer pectorals
When	Late in workout
Start	Lie back on a decline bench with your feet secured beneath the ankle pads. Hold a pair of dumbbells with the weights together and directly over your chest and your arms slightly bent.
Execution	Lower the weights down and out to the sides, maintaining just a slight bend in the elbows, until you feel a stretch in your chest. Contract your pectorals to return the dumbbells to the start position and squeeze the muscles hard at the top.
Variation	Decrease the angle of decline to nearly flat (parallel with the floor) to work the middle pectorals more while still emphasizing the lower chest.
Advanced Tip	If you prefer to use a significantly heavier weight, bend your elbows more than normal as you lower the dumbbells. The resulting motion is a cross between a press and a fly.
Substitutes	Decline cable fly, cable crossover, machine fly

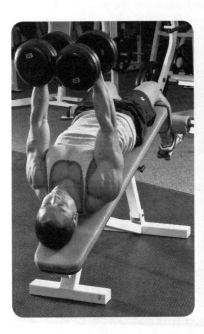
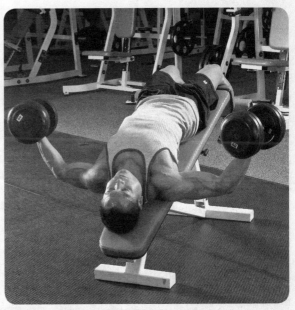

CABLE CROSSOVER

Target	Lower, inner, and outer pectorals
When	Late in workout
Start	Set the high pulleys on both sides of a cable station to above shoulder height and attach handles to them. Grab the handles, position yourself directly in the middle of the station, and step forward 1 to 2 feet (about 30 to 60 cm) so that the weights aren't resting on the stack. Begin with your arms extended out to your sides and your elbows slightly bent and pointed upward.
Execution	Keeping only a slight bend in your elbows, contract your pectorals to bring the handles together in a wide arc in front of your lower chest and upper abdominals. Bring your hands together (or cross your hands over one another so that your wrists touch to get a stronger contraction), then squeeze your pectorals together hard for a count. Slowly return the handles to the start position.
Variation	To target the upper pectorals, set the pulleys at the very bottom position and pull the handles up to around face level.
Advanced Tip	After touching your hands together or crossing them over at the top of the rep, push the handles out in front of you by further contracting your pectorals to extend your elbows.
Substitutes	Machine fly, cable fly, dumbbell fly—flat bench

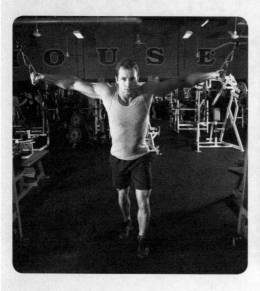 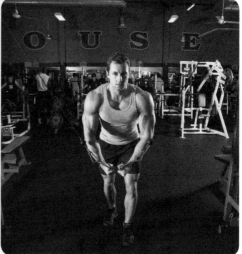

CHAPTER 5

Back Exercises

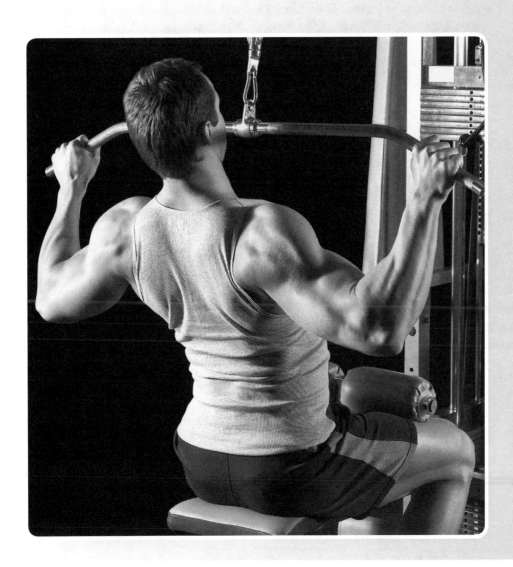

The two main types of back exercises are lat pull-downs or pull-ups (virtually the same motion) and rows. There are many variations of both types of exercises, as you'll see in this chapter. Pull-downs and pull-ups (wide-grip versions, at least) primarily develop width in the back by targeting the outer portions of the latissimus muscles; rows are ideal for creating thickness by building up such middle-back muscles as the rhomboids and middle trapezius. Both types of movements involve multiple joints and should typically be done before the few single-joint exercises that exist for the back, such as straight-arm pull-downs, pull-backs, and back extensions for the lower-back muscles.

As for which major exercise to perform first in your back workout—pull-downs and pull-ups or rows—it depends on your goals and weaknesses. If your primary objective is to increase back width, begin with a wide-grip pull-up or lat pull-down. Likewise, if your back lacks thickness, do your rows first. Otherwise, alternating between pull-downs or pull-ups and rows first is wise.

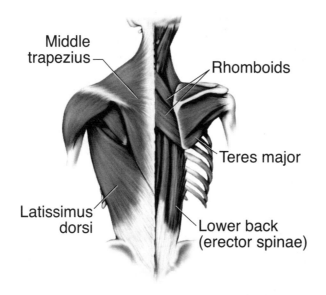

LAT PULL-DOWN

Target   Upper latissimus muscles

When   Early in workout

Start   Grasp a pull-down bar wider than shoulder width with an overhand grip and sit on the seat with your knees secured underneath the pads. Begin with your arms extended overhead and your torso erect.

Execution   Leading with your elbows, pull the bar down by contracting your back muscles until the bar clears chin level. Squeeze your shoulder blades together for a count at the bottom, then slowly return the bar to the start position.

Variation   Perform the lat pull-down by pulling the bar behind the head and touching it to the back of the neck. If you have shoulder problems, however, this is not recommended.

Advanced Tip   After reaching failure on pull-downs, extend the set by using a reverse grip (which allows you more strength) to get a few more reps before reaching failure again.

Substitutes   Pull-up—wide grip, assisted pull-up, Hammer Strength lat pull-down or other cambered machine lat pull-down

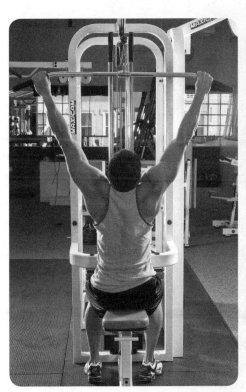 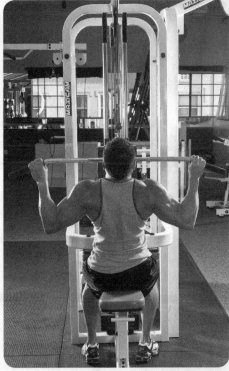

PULL-UP—WIDE GRIP

Target	Upper latissimus muscles
When	Early in workout
Start	Grasp a pull-up bar with an overhand grip just outside shoulder width. Begin by hanging straight down to the floor with your arms extended.
Execution	Contract your back muscles and bend your elbows to pull yourself straight up until your chin is over the bar. Slowly lower yourself to the start position.
Variation	Do this exercise behind the head. As you lift yourself up, lean forward slightly so that the back of your neck touches the bar at the top.
Advanced Tip	Achieve a full range of motion by touching your chest, not your chin, to the bar at the top of each rep.
Substitutes	Lat pull-down, assisted pull-up, Hammer Strength lat pull-down or other cambered machine lat pull-down

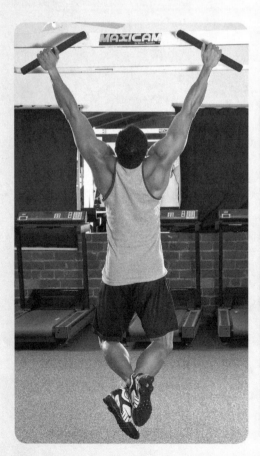 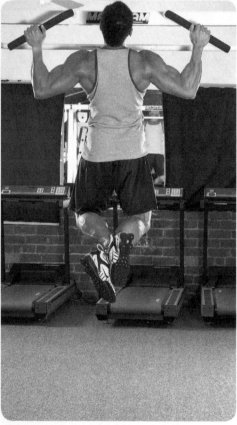

ASSISTED PULL-UP

Target	Upper latissimus muscles
When	Early in workout
Start	Select a weight that will assist you in reaching failure at your desired number of reps. Grasp the bar with a wide grip (outside shoulder width), then place your feet on the pegs. Lower yourself to an arms-extended position.
Execution	Pull yourself up, just as you would when doing a standard pull-up, until your chin reaches or passes the height of the bar. Squeeze your back muscles for a count, then slowly lower yourself back to the start position.
Variation	To target the lower latissimus muscles more, assume a narrow grip (either overhand or underhand) on the bar. Many assisted pull-up machines also include a neutral-grip option.
Advanced Tip	Combine body-weight pull-ups with assisted pull-ups by doing body-weight pull-ups to failure, then shift immediately to assisted pull-ups to reach a higher rep count. Eventually, you should be able to do more body-weight pull-ups.
Substitutes	Pull-up (wide grip or close grip), lat pull-down, Hammer Strength lat pull-down or other cambered machine lat pull-down

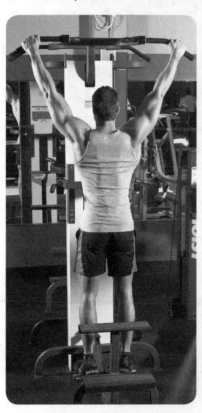 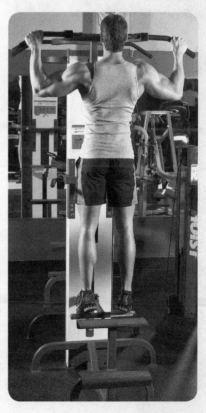

LAT PULL-DOWN–REVERSE GRIP

Target	Lower latissimus muscles
When	Middle to late in workout
Start	Grasp a pull-down bar with a narrow (hands 12 to 16 inches, or 30 to 40 cm, apart) underhand grip, and sit on the seat with your knees secured underneath the pads. Begin with your arms extended upward and your torso erect.
Execution	Leading with your elbows, pull the bar down by contracting your back muscles until the bar touches your upper chest. Squeeze your shoulder blades together for a count at the bottom, then slowly return the bar to the start position.
Variation	A narrow, neutral-grip handle (as you'd use for seated cable rows) can also target the lower latissimus muscles from a different angle.
Advanced Tip	To promote balance from side to side, perform the exercise one arm at a time by using a handle attachment instead of a bar.
Substitutes	Cambered machine or Hammer Strength lat pull-down using a narrow grip

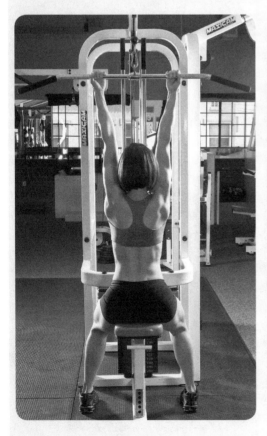 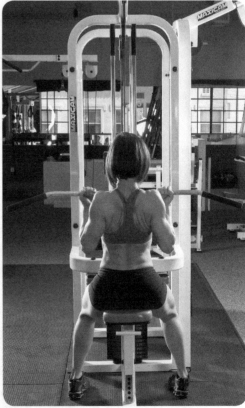

PULL-UP—CLOSE GRIP

Target	Lower latissimus muscles
When	Early in workout
Start	Grasp a pull-up bar with an inside shoulder-width overhand grip. Begin by hanging straight down to the floor with your arms extended.
Execution	Contract your back muscles and bend your elbows to lift yourself up until your chin is over the bar, keeping your lower body still throughout. Slowly lower yourself to the start position.
Variations	Perform this exercise with an underhand grip (commonly called a chin-up grip) or neutral grip. A neutral grip requires parallel pull-up bars, which look similar to dip bars.
Advanced Tip	A close-grip cable row attachment can be draped over the pull-up bar and used for neutral-grip pull-ups.
Substitutes	Lat pull-down—close grip, assisted pull-up (close grip), Hammer Strength lat pull-down (close grip)

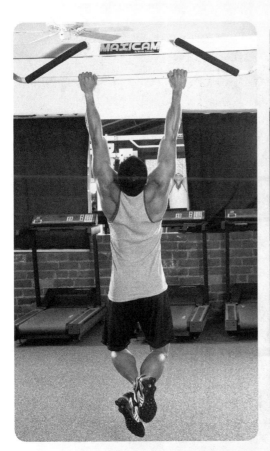 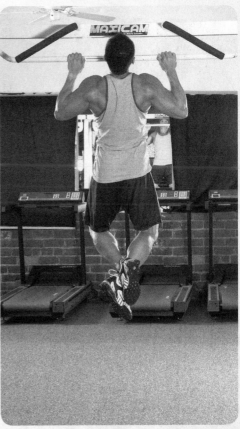

STRAIGHT-ARM CABLE PULL-DOWN

Target	Lower latissimus muscles
When	End of workout
Start	Stand facing a cable stack with a straight bar attached to the high pulley. Grasp the bar with a shoulder-width grip and step back a foot or two (about 30 to 60 cm) so the weight doesn't rest on the stack. Begin with your arms extended but not locked out, the bar at around head level, and a slight bend in your waist.
Execution	Keeping your arms extended, contract your back muscles to pull the bar down and toward you until it touches your thighs. Hold the contraction for a count, then slowly return the bar to the start position.
Variation	Use a rope attachment so that the hands are close together and in a neutral position (palms facing each other).
Advanced Tip	To extend the range of motion, bend farther at the waist so that your torso is at roughly a 45-degree angle to the floor. Begin each rep with your hands overhead.
Substitutes	Dumbbell, barbell, or machine pull-over

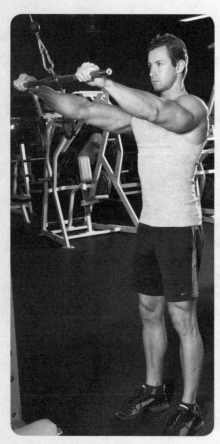
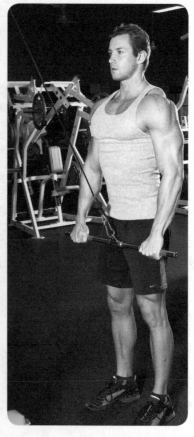

DUMBBELL STRAIGHT-ARM PULL-BACK

Target	Lower latissimus muscles
When	End of workout
Start	Stand while holding a light dumbbell in one hand with your knees slightly bent. Bend at the waist so that your torso is roughly parallel with the floor. Begin with your nonworking hand on the same-side knee for support and the working arm extended straight down toward the floor, palm facing back.
Execution	Contract your working-side lat muscle to pull the dumbbell back and up behind you, keeping your elbow extended. When your arm reaches a position parallel with the floor, slowly lower the dumbbell back to the start position.
Variations	For added support, you can perform this exercise with one knee and your nonworking hand on a flat bench, or, without the bench, with your nonworking hand holding onto a stable structure instead of resting on your knee.
Advanced Tip	Perform the pull-back with both arms simultaneously (each holding a light dumbbell); this requires more core stabilization.
Substitutes	Straight-arm cable pull-down, straight-arm pull-over

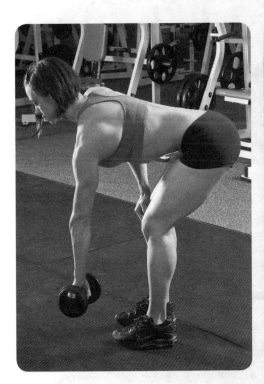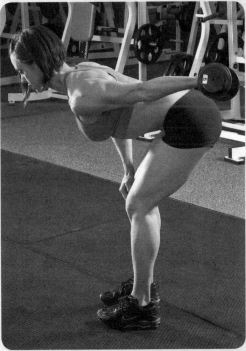

BARBELL BENT-OVER ROW

Target	Lower latissimus muscles, rhomboids, and middle trapezius
When	Early in workout
Start	Stand while holding a barbell with a shoulder-width overhand grip and your knees slightly bent. Bend at your waist so your torso is at or slightly above parallel to the floor. Start with the bar hanging straight down toward the floor and your arms extended.
Execution	Bend your elbows and contract your back muscles to pull the bar up to your abdomen, keeping your torso in the same position throughout. Squeeze the contraction at the top, then slowly lower the bar back to the arms-extended position.
Variation	Do this exercise with an underhand grip.
Advanced Tip	Going with a wider grip will target the upper latissimus, whereas using a narrow or underhand grip will focus on the lower latissimus. Choose your grip to improve your particular weakness, or vary the grips frequently for better overall back development.
Substitutes	Dumbbell bent-over row, Smith machine bent-over row

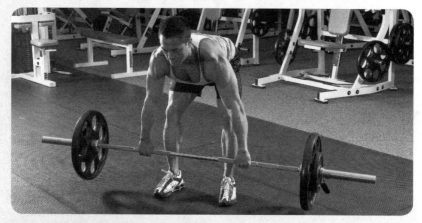

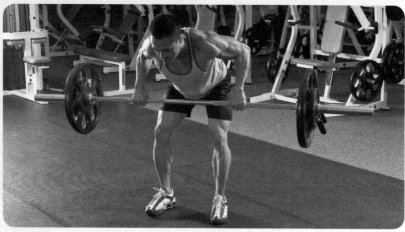

SMITH MACHINE BENT-OVER ROW

Target   Lower latissimus muscles, rhomboids, and middle trapezius

When   Early in workout

Start   Stand in the middle of a Smith machine and grasp the bar with a shoulder-width overhand grip. Unhook the releases, and bend at your waist so your torso is at about a 45-degree angle to the floor. Begin with your arms extended straight down toward the floor, your back flat, and your knees slightly bent.

Execution   Pull the bar up to your midsection by contracting your back muscles and bending your elbows. When the bar reaches your abdomen, squeeze your shoulder blades together, then slowly lower the bar to the start position.

Variations   Perform bent-over rows with an underhand grip to focus on the lower latissimus muscles.

Advanced Tip   Assume a wider grip to target the upper latissimus muscles or a narrow grip for the lower latissimus muscles. Choose your grip to improve your particular weakness, or vary the grips frequently for better overall back development.

Substitutes   Barbell bent-over row, dumbbell bent-over row

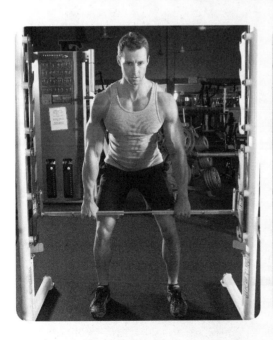
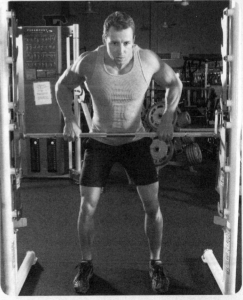

DUMBBELL BENT-OVER ROW

Target	Lower latissimus muscles, rhomboids, and middle trapezius
When	Early in workout
Start	Stand with your knees slightly bent while holding a pair of dumbbells. Bend at your waist so your torso is at or slightly above parallel to the floor, and start with the dumbbells hanging straight down toward the floor, with your palms facing each other and your arms extended.
Execution	Maintaining the same torso angle, pull the dumbbells up in unison until they reach waist height. Squeeze your shoulder blades together to achieve full contraction in the back muscles, then lower the weights to the start position.
Variations	To train the muscles from a slightly different angle, perform the motion with your palms facing forward or backward.
Advanced Tip	Begin each rep with your palms facing back; as you lift the dumbbells up, rotate your wrists so that by the top of the rep your palms are facing forward.
Substitutes	Barbell bent-over row, Smith machine bent-over row

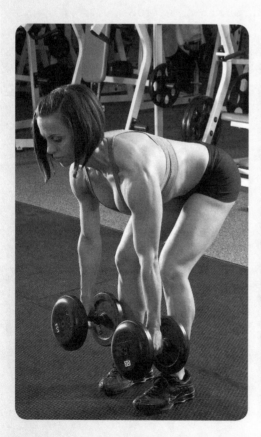
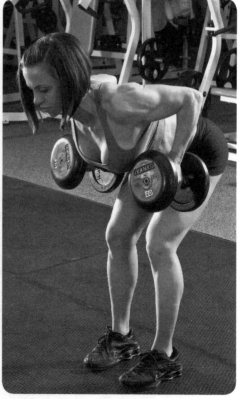

ONE-ARM DUMBBELL ROW

Target   Lower latissimus muscles, rhomboids, and middle trapezius

When   Early in workout

Start   Place one bent knee and the same-side hand on a flat bench. Place the opposite foot on the floor and hold a dumbbell in that hand, hanging straight toward the floor, with your arm extended and palm facing in. Bend at the waist, with your back parallel with the floor and your eyes facing the floor.

Execution   Keeping your chest pointed to the floor, pull the dumbbell up to your waist by contracting your back muscles and bending your elbow. When the dumbbell reaches your waist, squeeze your shoulder blades together, then slowly lower the dumbbell to the start position. Complete all reps with one arm, then switch arms.

Variation   Do this exercise without using a flat bench: Hold on to a stable structure (such as a pole or dumbbell rack) with your nonworking hand. Keep both feet on the floor with the same bend at the waist.

Advanced Tip   For a slightly different feel, as you pull the dumbbell up, turn your wrist so that at the top of the rep your palm faces forward.

Substitutes   Smith machine one-arm row, low pulley one-arm cable row, seated cable row (done with one arm), machine row (done with one arm)

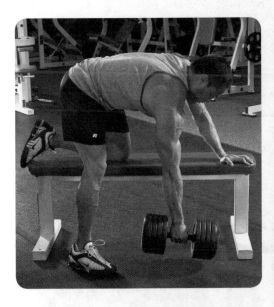
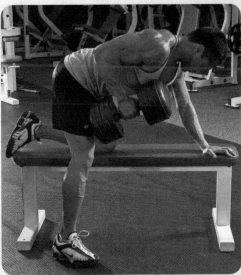

SMITH MACHINE ONE-ARM ROW

Target	Lower latissimus muscles, rhomboids, and middle trapezius
When	Early in workout
Start	Stand sideways to the bar and grasp the middle of it with your closer hand. Unhook the latches to release the bar. Begin with your knees slightly bent and your working arm extended toward the floor (your nonworking hand can be on your thigh or holding the machine to stabilize yourself). Bend over at the waist so your torso is at a 45-degree angle to the floor.
Execution	While keeping your torso still, pull the bar up as high as you can by contracting your back muscles and bending your elbow. Squeeze your shoulder blades together at the top, then slowly lower the bar back to the start position. Complete all reps with that arm, then switch arms.
Variation	For added stability, do this exercise with a flat bench (as with the one-arm dumbbell row), placing the bench parallel and close to the bar.
Advanced Tip	To develop more power and strength though ballistic training, pull the bar up as fast as you can without slowing it at the top. Let go of the bar when it reaches about waist level, then catch it on the way back down. Use a very light weight (a weight you can do about 20 to 25 normal reps with), but do no more than 8 reps in this manner, stopping well before reaching failure.
Substitutes	One-arm dumbbell row, low pulley one-arm cable row, seated cable row, machine row (done with one arm)

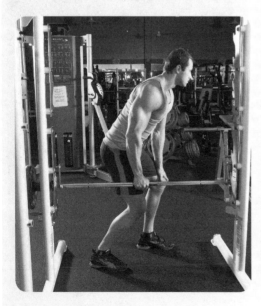 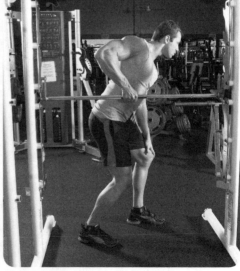

INCLINE DUMBBELL ROW

Target   Lower latissimus muscles, rhomboids, and middle trapezius

When   Middle of workout

Start   Lie facedown on an incline bench with your feet on the floor. Hold a pair of dumbbells. Begin with your arms hanging straight toward the floor, palms facing each other, and elbows fully extended.

Execution   Contract your back muscles and lead with your elbows to pull the dumbbells straight up. When they reach your midsection, squeeze your shoulder blades together for a count, then slowly lower the weights to the start position.

Variations   Start the movement with your palms facing forward, keeping them in this position as you perform the movement. Or begin with your palms facing each other, then turn them forward as you lift the weights.

Advanced Tip To train more stabilizing and core muscles, compromise your balance by bending your knees 90 degrees and placing them on the seat so that your feet are off the floor throughout.

Substitutes   Dumbbell bent-over row, Smith machine bent-over row, supported T-bar row

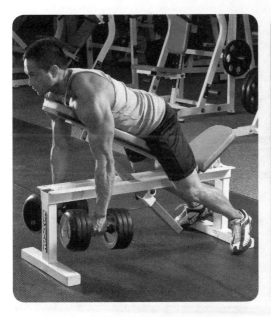 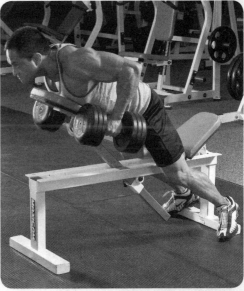

SEATED CABLE ROW

Target	Lower latissimus muscles, rhomboids, and middle trapezius
When	Early to middle of workout
Start	Sit upright at a cable row station with your feet in front of you on the platforms. Lean forward and grasp a narrow neutral-grip attachment. Begin with your arms extended out in front of you and your torso perpendicular to the floor. Keep your knees slightly bent and maintain the arch in your lower back.
Execution	Contract your back muscles and lead with your elbows to pull the handle in toward your midsection. When your hands reach your midriff, squeeze your shoulder blades together to achieve full contraction, then return the handle to the start position.
Variations	Perform cable rows with any number of handles and attachments, including a lat pull-down bar (take a wide grip to focus on the lower latissimus muscles for back width), a rope, or a wide neutral-grip bar.
Advanced Tip	For equal muscle development on both sides of the body, perform seated rows one arm at a time using a single handle.
Substitutes	T-bar row, machine row

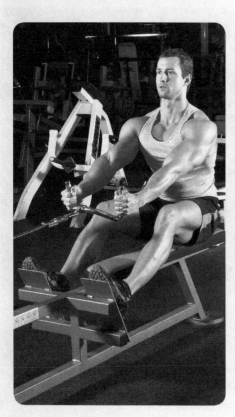 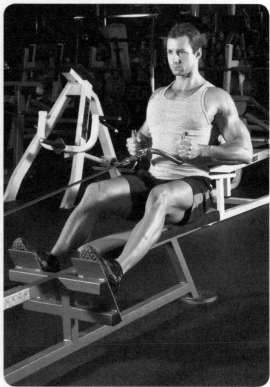

LOW PULLEY ONE-ARM CABLE ROW

Target   Lower latissimus muscles, rhomboids, and middle trapezius

When   Middle to late in workout

Start   Attach a handle to a low pulley cable, grasp the handle, and step back a foot or two (about 30 to 60 cm) so the weight doesn't rest on the stack. Begin with your knees slightly bent, your torso flat and at a 45-degree angle to the floor, your working arm extended down toward the floor (palm facing in), and your nonworking hand grasping the machine or on your thigh to stabilize yourself.

Execution   Contract your back muscles and bend your elbow to pull the handle up to your waist. When it reaches the waist, hold the contraction for a count, then slowly lower the handle back to the start position. Perform all reps with that arm, then switch arms.

Variations   Perform the cable row while one knee and one hand are on a flat bench (as with the one-arm dumbbell row, page 77) that is perpendicular to the weight stack.

Advanced Tip   As you pull the handle toward you, turn your wrist up so that by the top of each rep your palm and forearm are facing you.

Substitutes   One-arm dumbbell row, seated cable row (done with one arm)

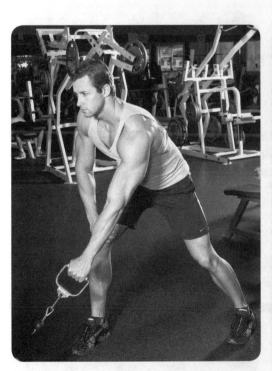 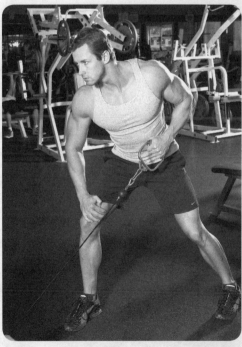

T-BAR ROW

Target	Lower latissimus muscles, rhomboids, and middle trapezius
When	Early in workout
Start	Stand on the platform with your feet roughly shoulder-width apart and knees slightly bent. Lean forward and grab the bar with a shoulder-width overhand grip, and begin with your arms extended below you and your torso about 45 degrees to the floor.
Execution	Pull the weight in toward you by contracting your back muscles and bending your elbows, keeping your chest out and lower back arched. At the top of the rep, squeeze your shoulder blades together, then slowly lower the weight back to the start position.
Variations	Most T-bar apparatuses offer multiple grip options (wide, narrow, neutral). Alternate grips every other workout, or even every other set, to train the back muscles from various angles.
Advanced Tip	The T-bar row is great for doing drop sets (see chapter 10, page 186) because the weight plates are at one end, which allows you to decrease weight quickly.
Substitutes	Seated cable row, supported T-bar row, barbell bent-over row

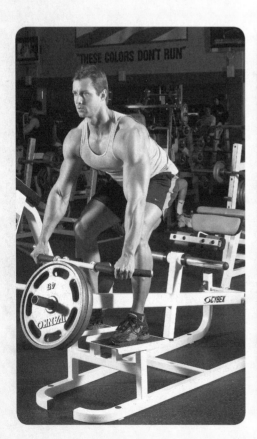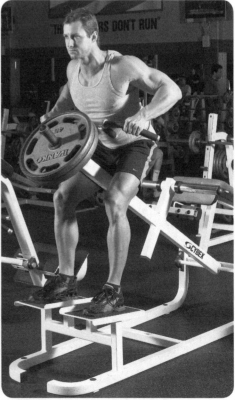

SUPPORTED T-BAR ROW

Target Lower latissimus muscles, rhomboids, and middle trapezius

When Early to middle of workout

Start Place your feet on the platform and your chest and abdomen on the angled pad. Grasp the bar with a shoulder-width grip, unrack it, and begin with your arms extended in front of you.

Execution Keeping your torso flush against the pad, pull the bar toward you by bending your elbows and contracting your back muscles. At the top of the motion, squeeze your shoulder blades together for full contraction, then slowly lower the bar back to the start position.

Variations As with unsupported T-bar rows, feel free to use any and all grip variations that the apparatus has to offer.

Advanced Tip Supported T-bar rows are also great for doing drop sets because you are able to decrease weight quickly.

Substitutes T-bar row, seated cable row, machine row

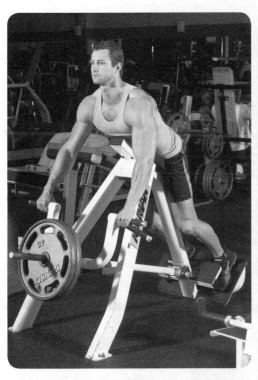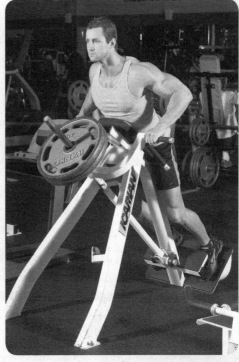

MACHINE ROW

Target	Lower latissimus muscles, rhomboids, and middle trapezius
When	Middle to late in workout
Start	Adjust the seat of a row machine so that in the top position the handles are at midriff height. Begin with your chest and abdomen touching the pad (if there is one), your feet flat on the floor, and your arms extended in front of you; hold on to the handles.
Execution	Pull the handles toward you as far as you can, keeping your chest and abdomen in contact with the pad. Squeeze your shoulder blades together for full contraction, then slowly return to the start position.
Variations	A variety of seated row machines, including Hammer Strength brand (pictured), generally target the same muscles. Feel free to use different machines when you have the opportunity to incorporate variety into your training.
Advanced Tip	To target the lower latissimus muscles, raise the seat higher so that you're pulling the handles to a lower point. To target the upper latissimus muscles, lower the seat so that you're pulling to your chest and use a wider grip if available.
Substitutes	Seated cable row, supported T-bar row

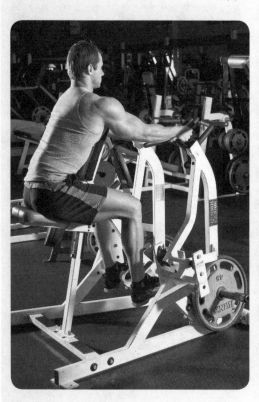 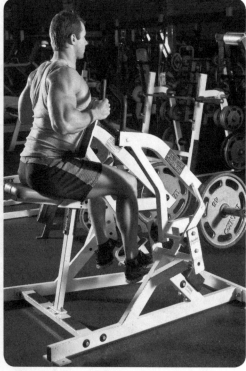

BACK EXTENSION

Target	Lower back
When	End of workout
Start	Adjust the apparatus so that the top of the leg pad is just below your waist. Secure your feet in front of the ankle pads and place your thighs against the thigh pads, with your legs straight. Begin with your upper body aligned with your lower body and your arms crossed over your chest.
Execution	Bend at the waist to lower your torso toward the floor. When your waist reaches roughly a 90-degree angle, contract your lower-back muscles to lift your torso back to the start position.
Variations	The leg pad and foot platforms on most back extension apparatuses are slanted at a 45-degree angle. You can perform the back extension on apparatuses on which the leg pad is parallel with the floor and in line with the ankle pads. Exercises on both versions are effective.
Advanced Tip	For added resistance, hold a weight plate against your chest while you perform the movement.
Substitutes	Back extension machine, lying back extension

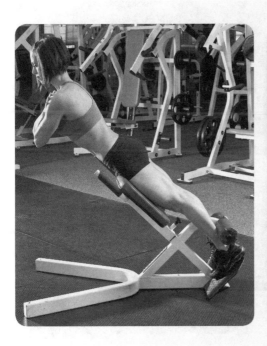
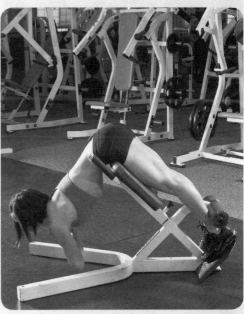

BACK EXTENSION MACHINE

Target	Lower back
When	End of workout
Start	Adjust the seat of the machine so that the padded arm rests on your upper back. Begin in an upright, seated position with your back against the pad. Use your hands to hold on to the pad for stability and begin with the weight off the stack.
Execution	Contract your lower-back muscles to push the pad back and lower your torso toward the floor in a slow, controlled manner as far down as the machine allows. Resist the weight to slowly raise your torso back up to the start position.
Variations	Various manufacturers make different versions of the back extension machine. Follow the instructions printed on each particular machine (if different from this description) to ensure proper technique.
Advanced Tip	After reaching failure, do a drop set, dropping 20 to 30 percent of the weight from the stack.
Substitutes	Back extension, lying back extension

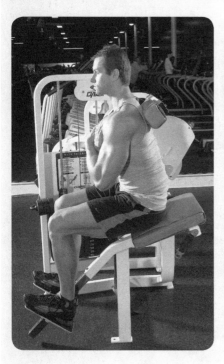
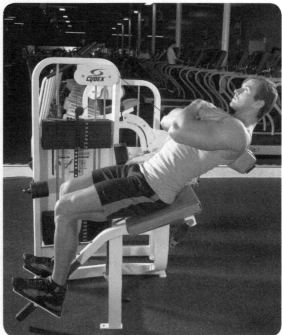

LYING BACK EXTENSION

Target	Lower back
When	End of workout
Start	Lie facedown on an open floor or mat with your arms extended out in front of you on the floor.
Execution	Contract your lower-back muscles to lift your arms and chest up off the floor as high as you can. The range of motion will be short. Squeeze your back muscles for a count, then slowly return to the start position without resting your head on the floor.
Variations	Raise your legs off the floor simultaneously with your chest and arms for additional lower-back stimulation as well as lower-body involvement. Extensions done this way are known as Supermans.
Advanced Tip	For added resistance, hold a light weight or a medicine ball in your extended arms as you perform the movement.
Substitutes	Back extension, back extension machine

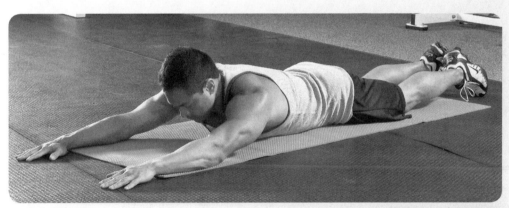

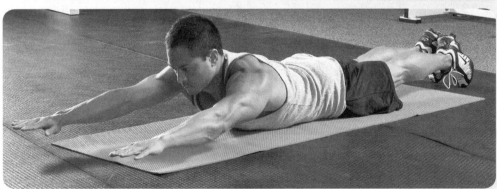

CHAPTER 6

Shoulder and Trapezius Exercises

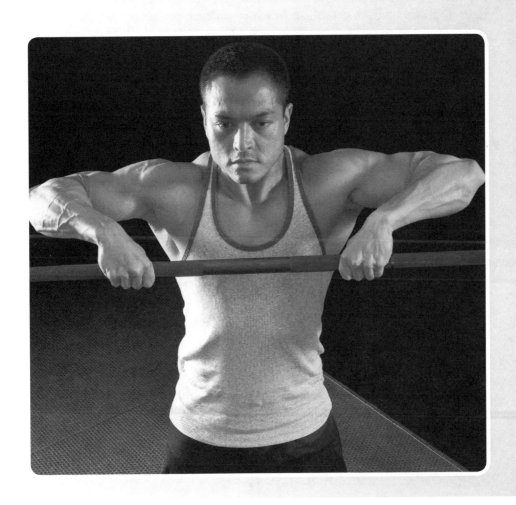

Shoulder training can be classified into exercises that train the deltoid muscles and exercises that train the upper trapezius muscles. The latter is a significantly smaller muscle group overall. Deltoid exercises are broken down into the three main types: overhead presses, upright rows, and raises. The first two types are compound exercises; you should perform them early in your workout. And because overhead presses typically allow you to use more weight for greater gains in muscular size and strength, in most situations you should do some version of them (barbell, dumbbell, or machine overhead press) first in your shoulder workout.

Raises isolate each of the three deltoid muscles: Front raises work the front deltoids, lateral raises train the middle deltoids, and bent-over (rear) raises work the rear deltoids. The decision on which type of raises you do first (after overhead presses or upright rows) depends on which of your deltoids deserves the most attention because of a relative weakness. If none of the three stands out as lagging behind, rotate the order among the three. Regardless, to promote balance in the shoulders, give all three deltoid groups ample attention in every workout.

Because the upper trapezius muscles are a significantly smaller muscle group than the deltoids, they should be trained after the deltoids. If your trapezius muscles are a significant weakness, train them on a different day than the deltoids, perhaps with an unrelated muscle group such as the legs or arms. The main exercise for trapezius is the shrug, a movement with a short range of motion that isolates the upper trapezius from the surrounding deltoids. Despite limited exercises for the trapezius, you can train shrugs using numerous variations, as you'll see near the end of this chapter.

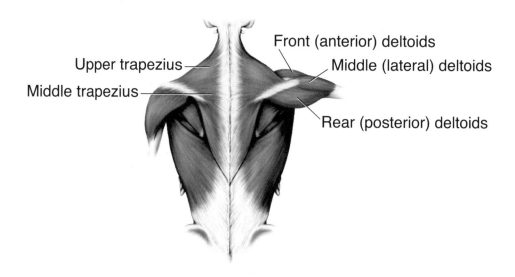

BARBELL OVERHEAD PRESS

Target	Middle and front deltoids
When	Early in workout
Start	Sit on an upright seat, using a rack if one is available, and grasp the bar with a wider-than-shoulder-width grip. Slowly lower the bar down in front of your face until it's below chin level.
Execution	Forcefully press the bar up and over your head without locking out your elbows at the top. Slowly lower the bar back to the start position.
Variation	Perform overhead presses behind the neck to deemphasize the front deltoids and involve more middle deltoids. Lower the bar behind your head to the point at which the barbell is even with the top of your ears.
Advanced Tip	Do overhead presses while standing, which requires using your whole body for stability. Keep a slight bend in the knees throughout, which will help relieve lower-back pain because your legs will absorb some of the force.
Substitutes	Dumbbell overhead press, Smith machine overhead press, machine overhead press

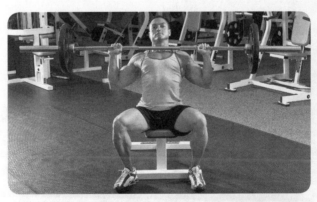

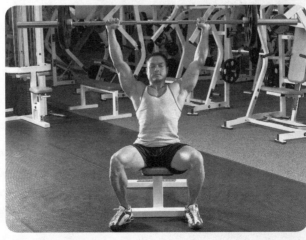

DUMBBELL OVERHEAD PRESS

Target	Middle and front deltoids
When	Early in workout
Start	Sit on a low-back seat or adjustable bench set upright while holding a pair of dumbbells. Lift the dumbbells up so you begin with them just outside your shoulders with palms facing forward.
Execution	Press the dumbbells straight up by contracting your shoulder muscles and extending your elbows until the weights are overhead, with your arms just short of locked out. Slowly lower the dumbbells to the start position.
Variation	To involve the front deltoids even more, perform the movement with your palms facing in (neutral grip) throughout.
Advanced Tip	As with the barbell overhead press, you can also perform this exercise while standing.
Substitutes	Barbell overhead press, Smith machine overhead press, machine overhead press

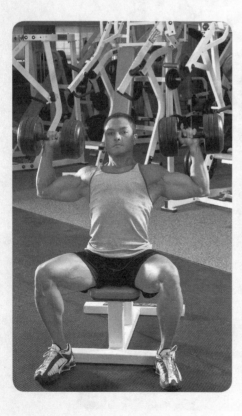 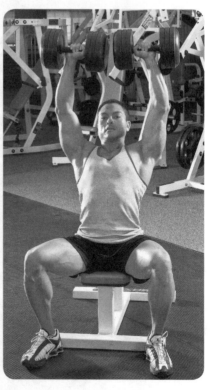

SMITH MACHINE OVERHEAD PRESS

Target   Middle and front deltoids

When   Early in workout

Start   Position a low-back seat, or an adjustable bench set upright, symmetrically in the middle of a Smith machine so that when you lower the bar it nearly touches your face. Sit on the seat or bench, grasp the bar with a wider-than-shoulder-width grip (palms forward), unhook the latches, and slowly lower the bar down in front of your face until it's below chin level.

Execution   Forcefully press the bar up and over your head without locking out your elbows at the top. Slowly lower the bar back to the start position.

Variations As with barbell overhead presses, you can perform this exercise behind the neck by moving the seat or bench up so that the bar lowers behind your head (this better emphasizes the middle deltoids). To target the front deltoids, move your hands slightly closer together (shoulder width) and use a reverse grip (palms facing you).

Advanced Tip To promote muscular balance, do the exercise one arm at a time, gripping the bar with your working hand outside of shoulder width and your nonworking hand on your hip to stabilize yourself. Use approximately half the weight of the two-arm version.

Substitutes Barbell overhead press, dumbbell overhead press, machine overhead press

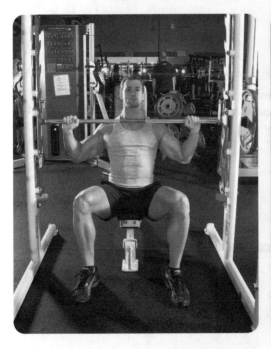
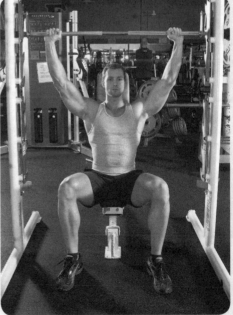

MACHINE OVERHEAD PRESS

Target — Middle and front deltoids

When — Early in workout

Start — Adjust the seat of an overhead press machine so that you are able to extend your arms at the top of the range of motion and can lower the handles down to your shoulders without the weight resting on the stack. Begin seated while holding on to the handles with your hands just outside your shoulders and your palms facing forward.

Execution — Contract your deltoids and extend your arms to press the handles straight up until your elbows are extended but not locked out. Slowly lower the weight back to the start position.

Variations — Most pressing machines offer various placements for your hands (wide, narrow, neutral, and reverse grip). Alter your grip occasionally to train the muscles from multiple angles.

Advanced Tip — To mimic a behind-the-neck press, sit backward on the seat (facing the seat back), and then use the same exercise technique.

Substitutes — Barbell overhead press, dumbbell overhead press, Smith machine overhead press

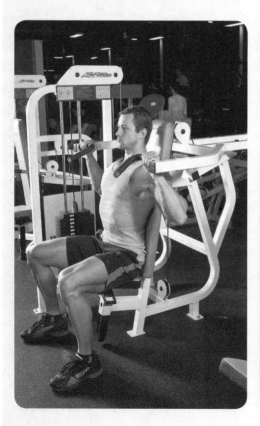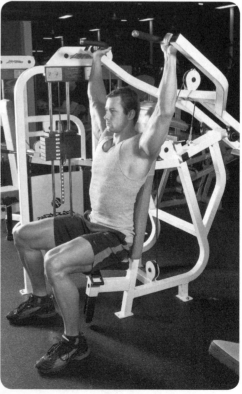

BARBELL UPRIGHT ROW

Target	Middle and front deltoids; upper trapezius
When	Early in workout, after overhead presses
Start	Stand while holding a barbell with an overhand shoulder-width grip down in front of you, with your arms extended. Keep a slight bend in your knees.
Execution	Without shrugging your shoulders (keep your shoulders depressed), contract your deltoids and bend your elbows to pull the bar up your body to chest height. Hold at the top for a count, then slowly lower the bar to the start position.
Variation	Some people find that using a straight bar aggravates the wrists; in this case, use an EZ-bar, which angles the wrists slightly inward for greater comfort.
Advanced Tip	Perform upright rows with a narrower grip (hands as close as 6 inches, or 15 cm, apart) to train the front deltoids and trapezius more, or use a very wide grip to target the middle deltoids more.
Substitutes	Dumbbell upright row, cable upright row, Smith machine upright row

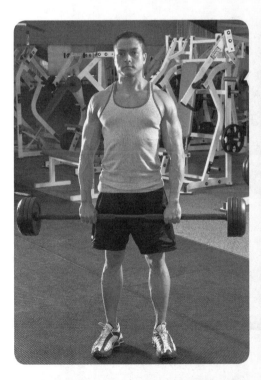 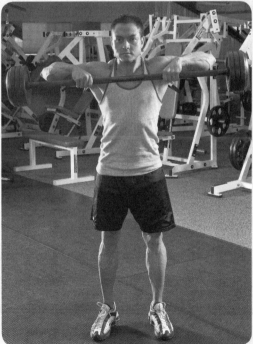

DUMBBELL UPRIGHT ROW

Target	Middle and front deltoids; upper trapezius
When	Early in workout, after overhead presses
Start	Stand while holding a pair of dumbbells in front of your thighs, with your arms extended and palms facing the front of your thighs. Maintain a slight bend in your knees.
Execution	Contract your deltoids and bend your elbows to pull both dumbbells up your body until your elbows point out to the sides and your upper arms are past parallel with the floor. Pause for a count, then slowly lower the weights back to the start position.
Variation	To work the middle deltoids more, begin with your hands farther apart so that the dumbbells are outside your thighs, not in front of them. From there, pull the weights straight up as high as you can.
Advanced Tip	Perform dumbbell upright rows one arm at a time; this requires more core stability.
Substitutes	Barbell upright row, cable upright row, Smith machine upright row

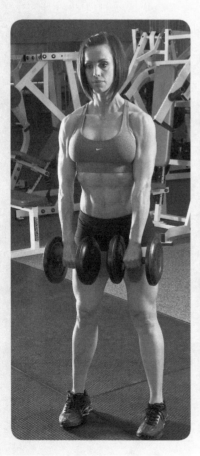
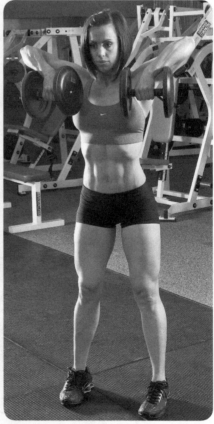

CABLE UPRIGHT ROW

Target	Middle and front deltoids; upper trapezius
When	Early in workout, after overhead presses
Start	Attach a straight bar to a low pulley cable. Stand while facing the stack and grasp the bar with a shoulder-width overhand grip. Begin with your arms extended toward the floor and your knees slightly bent.
Execution	Contract your deltoids and bend your elbows out to the sides to pull the bar up to chest level. Hold for a count at the top, then slowly return to the start position.
Variations	Use a lat pull-down bar for wide-grip upright rows; likewise, use an EZ-bar attachment to take pressure off the wrists.
Advanced Tip	To isolate each arm, perform the exercise unilaterally by attaching a handle to the low pulley.
Substitutes	Barbell upright row, dumbbell upright row, Smith machine upright row

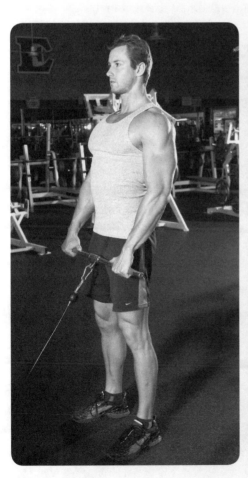 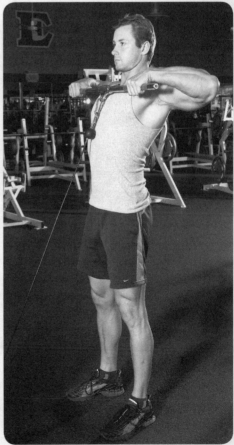

SMITH MACHINE UPRIGHT ROW

Target	Middle and front deltoids; upper trapezius
When	Early in workout, after overhead presses
Start	Set the bar of a Smith machine to a low placement. Grasp the bar with a shoulder-width overhand grip and begin while standing upright, with your arms extended toward the floor and your knees slightly bent.
Execution	Contract your deltoids and bend your elbows out to the sides to pull the bar straight up to chest level. Pause for a count, then slowly return the bar to the start position.
Variations	To train the middle deltoids more, use a wider grip; to involve the front deltoids and trapezius more, move your hands closer together.
Advanced Tip	Because the bar is set on a fixed path, you can also perform this exercise one arm at a time. Most modern Smith machines allow you to hold the bar off center so you can keep your hand placement the same.
Substitutes	Barbell upright row, dumbbell upright row, cable upright row

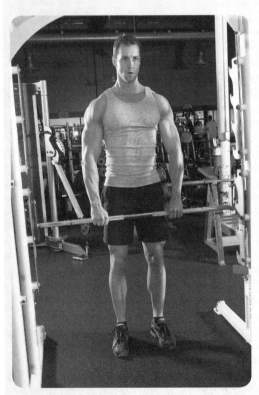 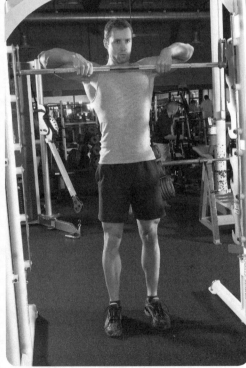

ARNOLD PRESS

Target   Front and middle deltoids (front deltoid emphasis)

When   Early in workout

Start   Sit on a low-back seat or adjustable bench set upright while holding a pair of dumbbells. Begin holding the weights in front of your shoulders with your palms facing you (supinated).

Execution   Press the dumbbells overhead while simultaneously pronating your wrists so that by the top of the rep your palms face forward. Slowly lower the dumbbells to the start position, rotating your wrists back in to the supinated position as you do so.

Variations   Alter the exercise either by not rotating your wrists (keeping your palms facing you) or by rotating only to neutral (palms facing each other).

Advanced Tip   Perform the exercise one arm at a time, holding on to the seat with your nonworking hand to stabilize yourself.

Substitutes   Smith machine overhead press (reverse grip), machine overhead press (reverse grip)

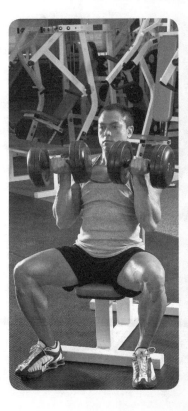 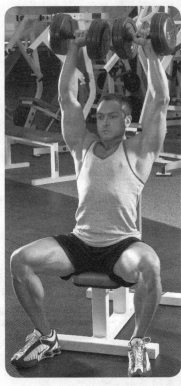

DUMBBELL LATERAL RAISE

Target	Middle deltoids
When	Middle to late in workout
Start	Stand while holding a pair of light dumbbells at your sides (palms facing in) with your elbows and knees slightly bent.
Execution	Maintaining only a slight bend in your elbows, raise the dumbbells up and out to the sides by contracting your deltoids. When your arms are about parallel with the floor, pause for a count, then slowly lower the dumbbells back to the start position.
Variations	Perform lateral raises while seated (using the same technique as standing) as well as one arm at a time.
Advanced Tip	For a stronger contraction, extend the range of motion by lifting your arms past parallel with the floor at the top; at the bottom, stop the dumbbells 6 to 12 inches (15 to 30 cm) short of your legs to keep constant tension on the deltoids and make the exercise more difficult.
Substitutes	Cable lateral raise, machine lateral raise

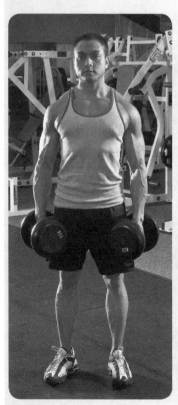
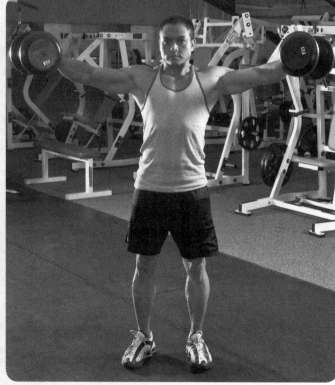

CABLE LATERAL RAISE

Target	Middle deltoids
When	Middle to late in workout
Start	Attach a handle to a low pulley cable. Stand sideways to the stack with knees slightly bent. Grab the handle with the hand that's farther away. Begin with your working elbow slightly bent and that hand almost touching your outer thigh. Place your nonworking hand on your hip or the machine to stabilize yourself.
Execution	While maintaining only a slight bend in the elbow, pull the handle up and out to the side by contracting your deltoids. When your arm is about parallel with the floor, pause and slowly return to the start position. Repeat for desired number of reps, then perform with the other arm.
Variations	Perform cable lateral raises two arms at a time by standing in the middle of a cable crossover station and holding a handle in each hand (hold the right-side handle in your left hand, and vice versa). Begin with your arms crossed in front of you.
Advanced Tip	Extend the range of motion past parallel at the top.
Substitutes	Dumbbell lateral raise, machine lateral raise

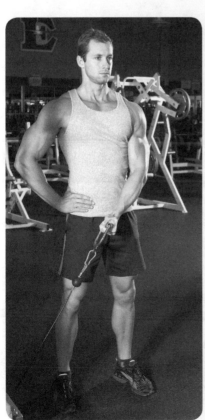
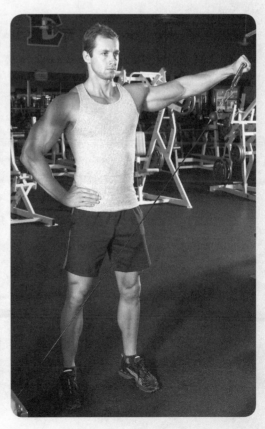

MACHINE LATERAL RAISE

Target	Middle deltoids
When	Late in workout
Start	Adjust the seat of the machine so that your forearms fit comfortably on the pads without causing you to shrug your shoulders. Begin with your elbows bent, arms on the pads, upper arms down at your sides, and the weight off the stack to provide tension.
Execution	Contract your deltoids to lift your arms up and out to the sides, keeping your forearms flush against the pads throughout. Hold at the top for a count, then slowly return to the start position.
Variations	Lateral raise machines vary depending on the manufacturer. Some have long arms with handles on the end, which allow you to keep your arms straight, more closely mimicking a dumbbell or cable lateral raise; others have pads like those pictured here. Most gyms have one or the other. If your gym has both, alternate between the two for variety.
Advanced Tip	Perform the movement while sitting backward on the machine to work the deltoids from a slightly different angle.
Substitutes	Dumbbell lateral raise, cable lateral raise

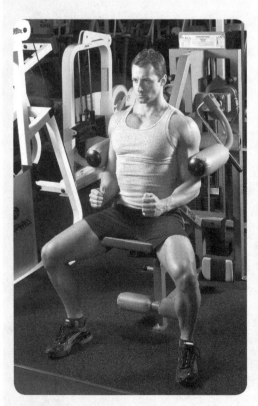 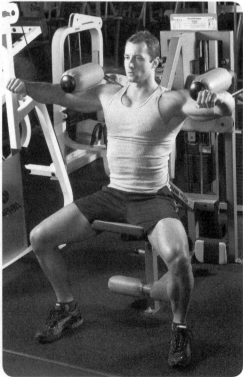

DUMBBELL FRONT RAISE

Target	Front deltoids
When	Late in workout
Start	Stand while holding a pair of dumbbells in front of your thighs with your arms extended toward the floor and your palms facing the front of your thighs. Bend your knees slightly.
Execution	With a slight bend in your elbow, raise one dumbbell up and out in front of you by contracting your front deltoid. When your arm is parallel with the floor, pause for a count, then return to the start position. Alternate arms every rep.
Variations	Perform front raises two arms at a time instead of in alternating fashion.
Advanced Tip	To increase the range of motion, continue lifting your arm past parallel until the dumbbell is directly overhead.
Substitutes	Barbell front raise, incline barbell front raise, prone incline barbell front raise, cable front raise

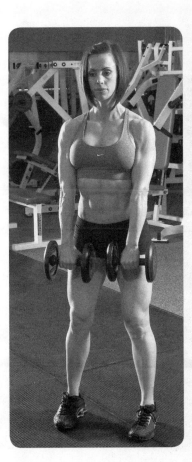 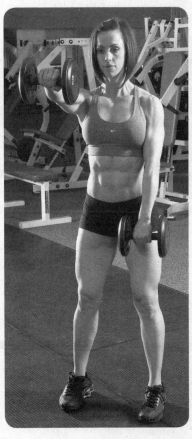

BARBELL FRONT RAISE

Target	Front deltoids
When	Late in workout
Start	Stand while holding a barbell in front of your thighs with a shoulder-width overhand grip and your arms extended toward the floor. Bend your knees slightly.
Execution	With a slight bend in your elbows, contract your front deltoids to lift the bar up and out in front of you until your arms are parallel with the floor. Hold the contraction for a count, then slowly return to the start position.
Variation	Instead of a barbell, use a weight plate, holding on to the sides of it with both hands. By the top of the rep, you should be looking directly at the plate's surface.
Advanced Tip	To keep constant tension on the front deltoids, stop the bar 6 to 12 inches (15 to 30 cm) short of your thighs at the bottom of each rep.
Substitutes	Dumbbell front raise, incline barbell front raise, prone incline barbell front raise, cable front raise

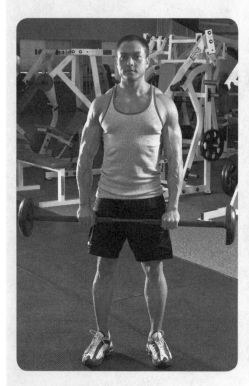 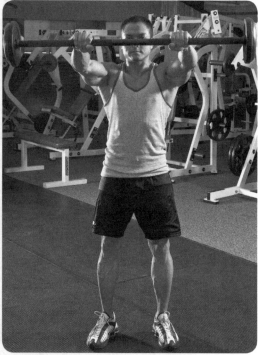

INCLINE BARBELL FRONT RAISE

Target   Front deltoids

When   Late in workout

Start   Lie back on an incline bench while holding a light barbell with a shoulder-width overhand grip. Begin with your arms extended but not locked out and the bar just above your thighs.

Execution   Keeping your elbows extended, contract your deltoids to lift the bar up until your arms are perpendicular to the floor. Slowly lower the weight to the start position without letting the bar rest on your legs at the bottom.

Variation   Perform this exercise while using dumbbells.

Advanced Tip   If using dumbbells, perform the exercise with your palms facing each other (neutral) to train the front deltoids from a slightly different angle.

Substitutes   Dumbbell front raise, barbell front raise, prone incline barbell front raise, cable front raise

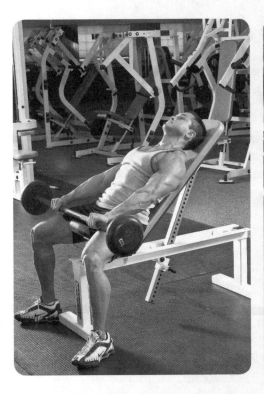 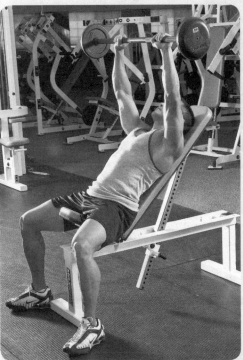

PRONE INCLINE BARBELL FRONT RAISE

Target

Front deltoids

When

Late in workout

Start

Lie facedown (prone) on an incline bench with your knees bent and your feet on the floor behind you. Grab a light barbell with a shoulder-width overhand grip and begin with it hanging straight toward the floor, arms extended.

Execution

Keeping your elbows extended but not locked out, lift the bar up and out in front of you until your arms are parallel with the floor. Slowly lower the bar to the start position.

Variation

Perform this exercise while using dumbbells.

Advanced Tip

To make the exercise more difficult, don't lower the bar all the way to where your arms are perpendicular to the floor; stop 6 to 12 inches (15 to 30 cm) short of that point at the bottom of each rep.

Substitutes

Dumbbell front raise, barbell front raise, incline barbell front raise, cable front raise

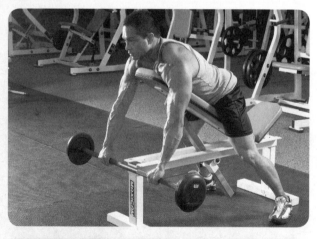

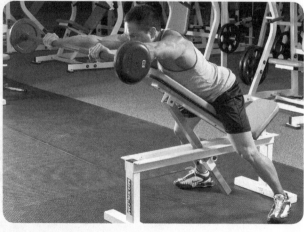

CABLE FRONT RAISE

Target	Front deltoids
When	Late in workout
Start	Attach a straight bar to a low pulley cable and stand close to but facing away from the weight stack. Grab the bar with a shoulder-width grip and run the cable between your legs. Begin with the bar just in front of your thighs with your arms extended but not locked out.
Execution	Keeping your arms straight, contract your front deltoids to lift the bar up in front of you until your arms are about parallel with the floor. Slowly lower to the start position.
Variation	Perform this one arm at a time by using a handle attachment. In this case, the cable should be to your side.
Advanced Tip	On the one-arm version, extend the range of motion by going past parallel at the top of each rep (this won't work on the two-arm version because the cable will be impeded).
Substitutes	Dumbbell front raise, barbell front raise, incline barbell front raise, prone incline barbell front raise

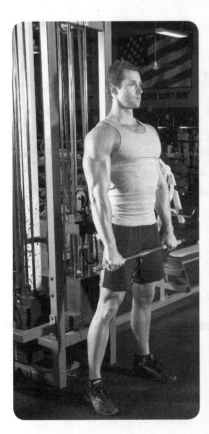 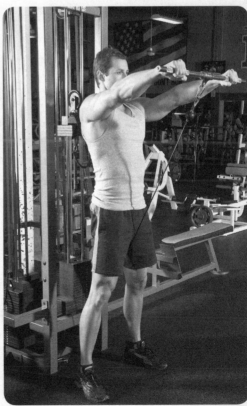

DUMBBELL BENT-OVER LATERAL RAISE

Target	Rear deltoids
When	Late in workout
Start	Hold a pair of dumbbells and bend over at the waist at a 45- to 90-degree angle with your back flat. Begin with the dumbbells hanging straight toward the floor, palms facing each other, and elbows extended.
Execution	With only a slight bend in the elbows, contract your rear deltoids to lift the weights out and up until your upper arms are roughly parallel with the floor. Hold the contraction for a count, then slowly lower to the start position.
Variation	Do this exercise while seated on a flat bench or seat by leaning forward so your chest is nearly touching your thighs. Keep your back flat and begin the motion with the dumbbells together under your thighs.
Advanced Tip	As you raise the dumbbells, rotate your wrists so that by the top of the movement your palms face back.
Substitutes	Cable bent-over lateral raise, cable reverse fly, machine reverse fly, cross-body rear deltoid raise

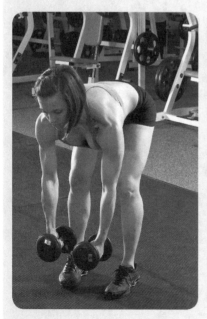
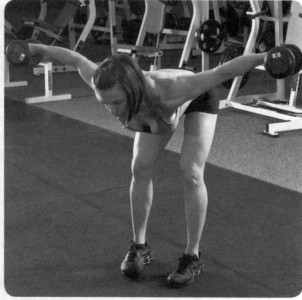

CABLE BENT-OVER LATERAL RAISE

Target   Rear deltoids

When   Late in workout

Start   Attach a handle to a low pulley cable, stand sideways to the weight stack, and grab the handle with the hand that's farther away. Bend over at the waist so that your torso is at a 45- to 90-degree angle to the floor. Begin with your working arm extended toward the floor (palm facing in) and your nonworking hand holding on to the machine or on your hip or thigh to stabilize yourself.

Execution   While keeping only a slight bend in your working elbow, contract your rear deltoid to lift the handle out and up in an arc until your arm is parallel with the floor. Slowly lower the handle to the start position. Perform all reps with that arm, then switch arms.

Variation   Perform this exercise with two arms at a time by positioning yourself in the middle of a cable crossover station and holding a handle in each hand (hold the right-side handle in your left hand, and vice versa). Begin with your arms crossed in front of you and bent over as described previously.

Advanced Tip   To alter the angle of pull slightly, perform the exercise with your palm facing behind you throughout. Do this by holding on to the cable directly (not attaching a handle to it) with your palm above the rubber stopper.

Substitutes   Dumbbell bent-over lateral raise, cable reverse fly, machine reverse fly, cross-body rear deltoid raise

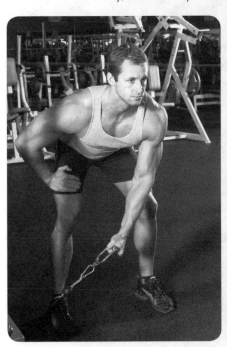 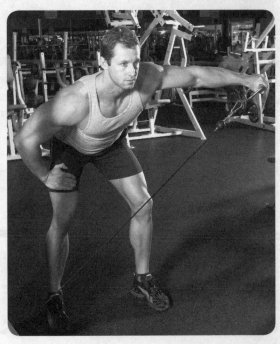

CABLE REVERSE FLY

Target	Rear deltoids
When	Late in workout
Start	Position two pulleys with handles attached at a cable crossover station just above shoulder height. With your right hand, grab the left-side handle, and vice versa, and stand in the middle of the station. Begin with your hands over your shoulders and elbows slightly bent.
Execution	Contract your rear deltoids to pull your arms out and to the sides, maintaining only a slight bend in the elbows, until your arms are in line with your back. Hold the contraction for a count, then slowly return to the start position.
Variation	Perform this exercise one arm at a time by standing closer to one side and holding on to the machine with your nonworking hand. Begin with the arm farther away from the stack in front of your chest.
Advanced Tip	For a slightly different angle of pull, move the pulleys up or down on the column and pull the handles up or down to shoulder height.
Substitutes	Dumbbell bent-over lateral raise, cable bent-over lateral raise, machine reverse fly, cross-body rear deltoid raise

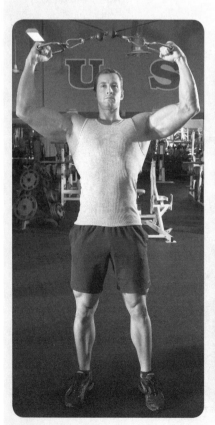
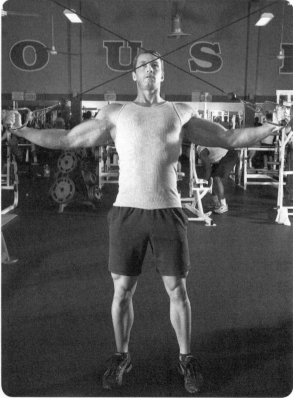

MACHINE REVERSE FLY

Target	Rear deltoids
When	Late in workout
Start	Adjust the seat of the machine (which likely doubles as a chest fly) so that when you hold on to the handles your hands are at shoulder height. Sit facing the machine and begin by holding on to the handles, with your arms extended in front of you.
Execution	Keeping your elbows straight but not locked out, contract your rear deltoids to pull the handles out and back until your arms are in line with your back. Hold the contraction for a count, then slowly return to the start position.
Variations	Many fly machines offer multiple grip options. Alternate between a neutral (palms facing each other) grip and a pronated (palms facing the floor) grip to train the rear deltoids from various angles.
Advanced Tip	To concentrate on each rear deltoid individually, perform this exercise one arm at a time.
Substitutes	Dumbbell bent-over lateral raise, cable bent-over lateral raise, cable reverse fly, cross-body rear deltoid raise

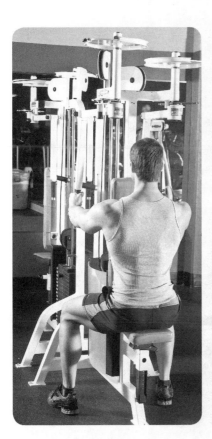 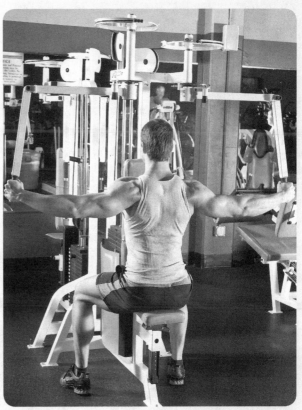

CROSS-BODY REAR DELTOID RAISE

Target	Rear deltoids
When	Late in workout
Start	Lie on your side on a flat bench while holding a light dumbbell in the opposite hand. Begin with the working arm across your chest (elbow extended), the dumbbell hanging toward the floor, and your nonworking arm on the bench.
Execution	Keeping your elbow extended but not locked out and your palm facing down, contract your rear deltoid to lift the dumbbell straight up until your arm is perpendicular to the floor. Hold the contraction for a count, then slowly lower to the start position. Perform all reps with that arm, then switch arms.
Variation	Instead of using a bench, lie sideways on an exercise ball to put more stabilizing muscles to work.
Advanced Tip	As you lift the dumbbell up, turn your pinky finger toward the ceiling so that by the top of the rep your palm faces your feet.
Substitutes	Dumbbell bent-over lateral raise, cable bent-over lateral raise, cable reverse fly, machine reverse fly

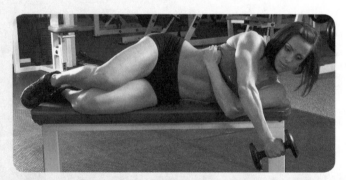

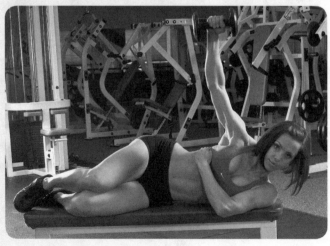

BARBELL SHRUG

Target	Upper trapezius
When	End of workout, after training deltoids
Start	Stand while holding a barbell in front of your thighs in a shoulder-width overhand grip. Bend your knees slightly.
Execution	While keeping your arms extended, elevate (shrug) your shoulders straight up (don't roll them back) as high as possible. Hold the contraction for a count, then depress your shoulders to lower the bar back to the start position.
Variation	Perform this exercise with the bar behind you. This helps keep your shoulders back and your chest out.
Advanced Tip	Spread your hands out wider than shoulder width to create a slightly different line of pull.
Substitutes	Dumbbell shrug, Smith machine shrug, prone incline dumbbell shrug, cable shrug

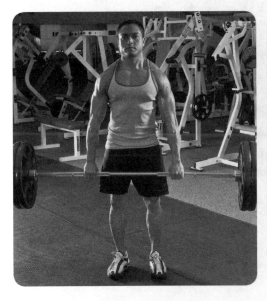 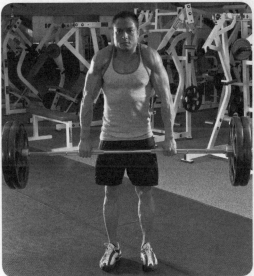

DUMBBELL SHRUG

Target	Upper trapezius
When	End of workout, after training deltoids
Start	Stand while holding a pair of dumbbells at your sides with your arms extended and your palms facing in. Bend your knees slightly.
Execution	While keeping your arms straight and hanging down toward the floor, shrug your shoulders straight up as high as possible. Hold the contraction for a count, then lower back to the start position.
Variation	To ensure you don't use your legs to help get the weight up, perform dumbbell shrugs while seated on a bench or seat.
Advanced Tip	To concentrate on each side individually, shrug one dumbbell up at a time while holding both dumbbells. Or perform the exercise with one dumbbell only, which also helps to build core strength.
Substitutes	Barbell shrug, Smith machine shrug, prone incline dumbbell shrug, cable shrug

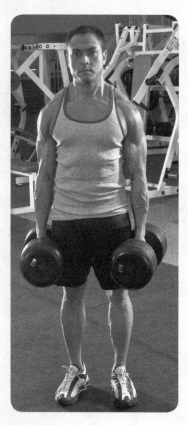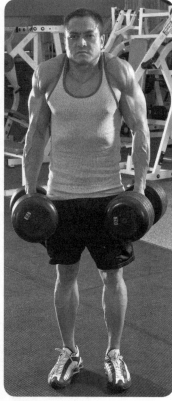

SMITH MACHINE SHRUG

Target	Upper trapezius
When	End of workout, after training deltoids
Start	Set the bar of a Smith machine at around knee level on the safety hooks. Grasp the bar with a shoulder-width overhand grip and stand up with it. Begin with your arms extended toward the floor, your knees slightly bent, and the bar just in front of your thighs.
Execution	Keeping the rest of your body stationary, shrug your shoulders straight up as high as possible. Hold the contraction for a count, then lower the bar back to the start position.
Variation	As with the barbell shrug, perform this exercise with the bar behind you. If your backside gets in the way as you lift the bar, simply move your feet forward—because the bar is supported by the guide rods of the machine, you can do this easily.
Advanced Tip	Do the exercise one arm at a time by turning sideways and grabbing the middle of the bar with one hand. Place your other hand either on your hip or on the machine to stabilize yourself. This helps you simultaneously build greater core strength and work your trapezius.
Substitutes	Barbell shrug, dumbbell shrug, prone incline dumbbell shrug, cable shrug

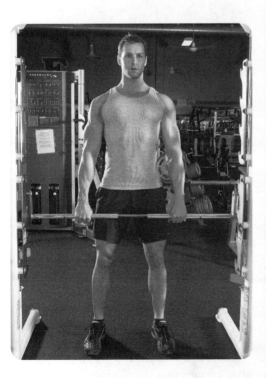
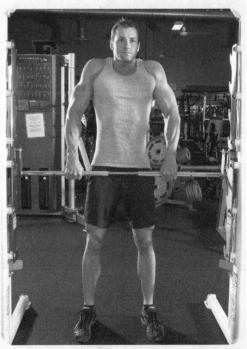

CABLE SHRUG

Target	Upper trapezius
When	End of workout, after training deltoids
Start	Stand in front of a cable stack with a straight bar attached to the low pulley. Grasp the bar with a shoulder-width grip and stand up straight with your arms extended toward the floor and the bar in front of your thighs.
Execution	With your arms extended, shrug your shoulders up toward the ceiling as high as possible. Hold at the top for a count, then return to the start position.
Variations	Perform cable shrugs with the bar behind the back by simply turning around and holding it behind you. You can also do them one arm at a time using a handle attachment.
Advanced Tip	Attach a handle to either side of a cable crossover station (on the low pulleys) and hold the handles while standing in the middle of the station. Shrug your shoulders up from there. This provides a line of pull toward the center of your body as well as up toward the ceiling.
Substitutes	Barbell shrug, dumbbell shrug, Smith machine shrug, prone incline dumbbell shrug

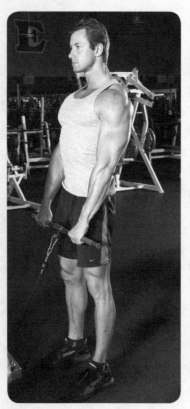 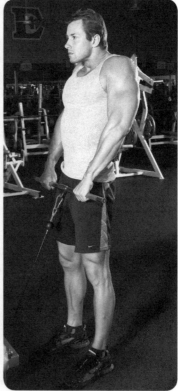

PRONE INCLINE DUMBBELL SHRUG

Target	Upper and middle trapezius
When	End of workout, after training deltoids
Start	Lie facedown on an incline bench set to approximately 45 degrees with the balls of your feet on the floor behind you. Grasp a pair of dumbbells and begin with your arms hanging straight down toward the floor and your palms facing each other.
Execution	Keeping your arms extended, shrug your shoulders straight up as high as possible. Hold at the top for a count, then slowly lower the dumbbells to the start position.
Variation	As with standard dumbbell shrugs, perform these one arm at a time in an alternating fashion—for each rep, shrug one side up and down, then do the other side.
Advanced Tip	Alter the angle of the bench to work various areas of the trapezius. Higher than 45 degrees will hit more of the upper trapezius and less of the middle trapezius; lower than 45 degrees will hit more of the middle trapezius and less of the upper trapezius.
Substitutes	Barbell shrug, dumbbell shrug, Smith machine shrug, cable shrug

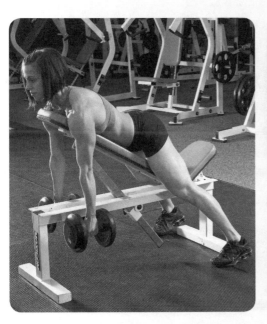 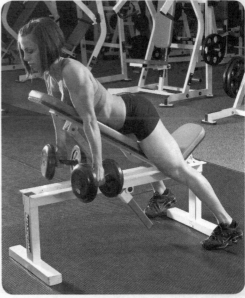

CHAPTER 7

Triceps Exercises

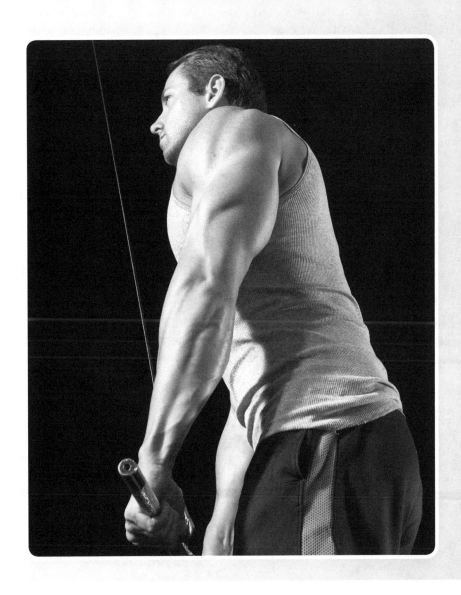

The majority of triceps exercises are isolation movements; the most notable exception is close-grip bench presses, a mass-building exercise for the back of the arms that you should do at the beginning of your triceps routine on days you include it. Isolation exercises for the triceps involve one common anatomical movement: elbow extension. Yet many arm positions (such as arms in front of you, behind you, and overhead) emphasize different heads of the triceps (long head, lateral head, and medial head), so exercises abound.

If there's one tip that applies to virtually every triceps exercise in terms of technique, it's that to truly isolate the muscle and minimize the involvement of surrounding muscles such as the chest and deltoids, you need to keep the elbows in as tight as possible, regardless of arm position. Allowing them to flare out will, in most cases, reduce the effectiveness of the exercise.

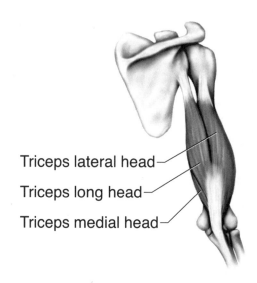

Triceps lateral head

Triceps long head

Triceps medial head

BARBELL BENCH PRESS—CLOSE GRIP

Target	Triceps lateral head
When	Early in workout
Start	Lie back on a flat bench with a rack and grasp a barbell at shoulder width with your palms facing forward. Unrack the bar and begin with it over your chest, your arms extended.
Execution	While keeping your elbows in tight to your body, slowly lower the bar down to your lower pectorals by bending your arms. When it touches, forcefully press the bar back up to the start position.
Variation	Perform close-grip bench presses on an incline or decline bench to train the triceps from a slightly different angle.
Advanced Tip	Press the bar straight up, not back toward your head as in regular bench presses—this will keep maximum tension on the triceps.
Substitute	Smith machine bench press—close grip

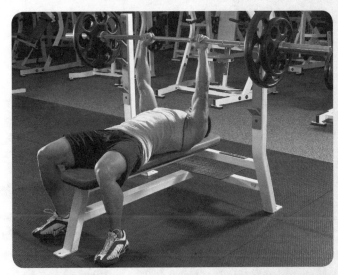

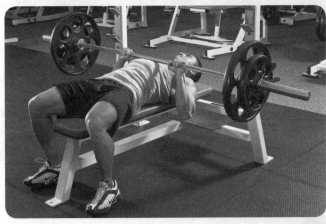

SMITH MACHINE BENCH PRESS—CLOSE GRIP

Target	Triceps lateral head
When	Early in workout
Start	Place a flat bench in a Smith machine so that the bar will touch your lower pectoralis at the bottom of each rep. Begin by lying back on the bench with the bar unhooked directly over your chest, your hands at shoulder width (palms facing forward), and your arms extended.
Execution	While keeping your elbows in at your sides, slowly lower the bar until it touches your lower chest. Forcefully press the bar back to the start position and squeeze your triceps for a count at the top to achieve full contraction.
Variations	As with the barbell close-grip press, you can also perform this exercise using an incline or decline bench.
Advanced Tip	To target the triceps medial head, use a reverse grip (palms facing back). This might require taking a slightly wider grip to relieve pressure on the wrists.
Substitute	Barbell bench press—close grip

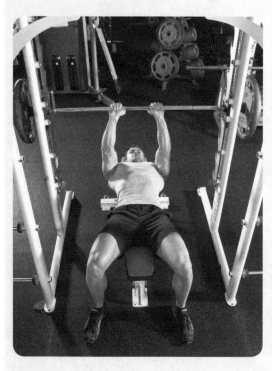 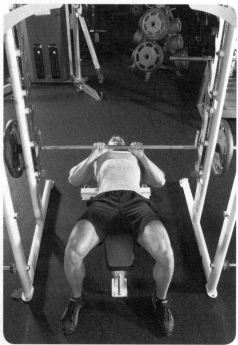

PUSH-UP—NARROW HAND POSITION

Target	Triceps lateral head
When	Late in workout, or when you have no other equipment
Start	Place your hands inside shoulder-width apart on the floor with your body flat and rigid and your toes on the floor. Begin with your arms extended, perpendicular to the floor.
Execution	Bend your elbows to slowly lower yourself down toward the floor. When your chest touches your hands, extend your elbows to press back up to the start position.
Variations	Push-up bars, which help keep your wrists flatter and allow you to use a neutral grip (palms facing each other), are available at some gyms and are for sale at fitness and sporting goods retailers. Some people find that push-up bars help relieve stress on the wrists.
Advanced Tip	A more difficult version is the diamond push-up, in which you form a diamond shape with your thumbs and index fingers on the floor for an even narrower hand placement and greater emphasis on the triceps.
Substitute	Barbell bench press—close grip

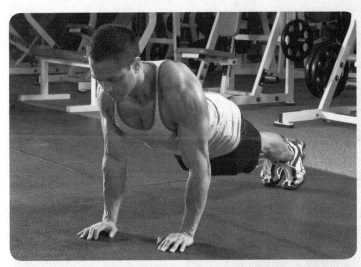

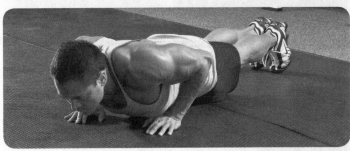

CABLE PRESS-DOWN

Target	Triceps lateral head
When	Early to middle of workout
Start	Attach a straight bar to a high pulley cable. Stand facing the weight stack and grab the bar with a shoulder width, overhand grip. Begin with your forearms just above parallel with the floor and your elbows in close to your sides.
Execution	Keeping your elbows in, contract your triceps to extend your elbows until your arms are straight. At the bottom, squeeze your triceps for a count, then slowly raise your hands back to the start position.
Variations	Use any number of attachments—EZ-bar, V-bar, rope—for this exercise to alter the angle of the movement. You can do cable press-downs one arm at a time with a handle attachment.
Advanced Tip	When using the rope attachment, at the bottom of each rep, turn your wrists out and squeeze hard to achieve full triceps contraction.
Substitutes	Barbell bench press—close grip, Smith machine bench press—close grip, decline lying barbell extension, triceps kickback

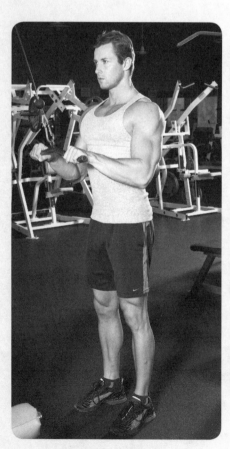 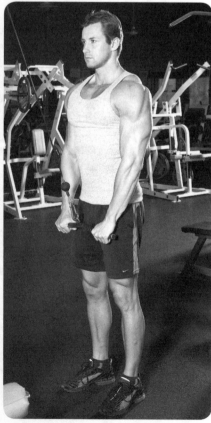

DUMBBELL KICKBACK

Target	Triceps lateral head
When	Late in workout
Start	Hold a dumbbell in one hand and place the same-side foot on the floor. Place your opposite knee and hand on a flat bench, and bend at the waist so your torso is parallel with the floor. Begin with your working arm bent at roughly 90 degrees, your upper arm parallel with the floor, palm facing in, and your elbow in tight against your body.
Execution	Keeping your upper arm stationary, contract your triceps to extend your elbow until your entire arm is parallel with the floor. Squeeze the contraction hard at the top with your elbow locked out, then lower the dumbbell to the start position.
Variation	Perform this exercise two arms at a time. Bend over at your waist so your torso is parallel with the floor instead of using a bench. Keep both upper arms parallel with the floor and your elbows in tight throughout.
Advanced Tip	As you extend your elbow, turn your wrist back so that by the top of the rep your palm faces the ceiling.
Substitutes	Cable kickback, cable press-down

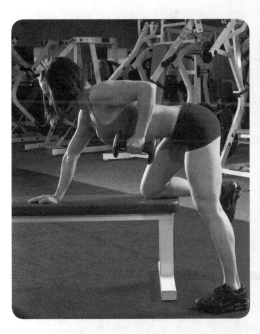 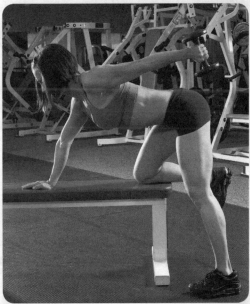

CABLE KICKBACK

Target	Triceps lateral head
When	Late in workout
Start	Stand in front of a low pulley cable with no bar or handle attached to it. Grab the cable cord just below the rubber stopper (palm facing in) and bend over at your waist so that your torso is between 45 degrees and parallel with the floor. Stagger your feet slightly for balance and begin with your working arm bent at 90 degrees, your upper arm parallel with the floor, and your elbow in tight to your body. Place your nonworking hand on your knee for support.
Execution	While keeping your upper arm stationary, contract your triceps to extend your elbow until your arm is locked out. Squeeze the contraction for a count, then return to the start position.
Variations	Use a rope attachment (hold both ends of the rope in your working hand) if you'd rather not hold on to the cable. You can also perform this exercise with a reverse grip, using a D-handle, to work more of the medial head.
Advanced Tip	As with the dumbbell kickback, as you extend your elbow, turn your wrist to face the ceiling by the top of the rep.
Substitutes	Dumbbell kickback, cable press-down

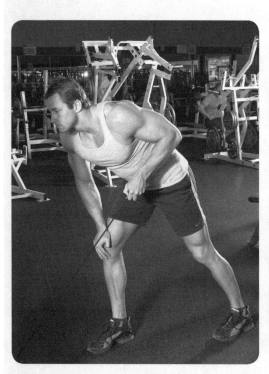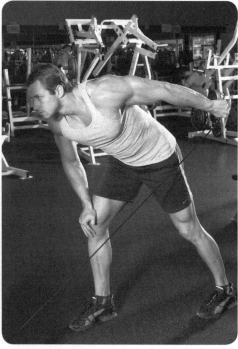

DECLINE LYING BARBELL EXTENSION

Target	Triceps lateral head
When	Early in workout
Start	Lie back on a decline bench while holding a barbell with a shoulder-width overhand grip. Begin with your arms extended straight up toward the ceiling and the bar directly over your chest.
Execution	While keeping your elbows in and your upper arms stationary, lower the bar down to your forehead. When it touches, extend your elbows to press the bar back to the start position.
Variations	Perform this exercise with either an EZ-bar or dumbbells.
Advanced Tip	From set to set, vary the degree of decline slightly (up or down) to train the triceps from a variety of angles.
Substitutes	Lying barbell extension, lying dumbbell extension, lying cable extension (decline variation), cable press-down

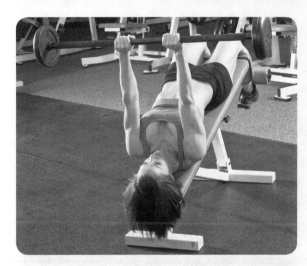

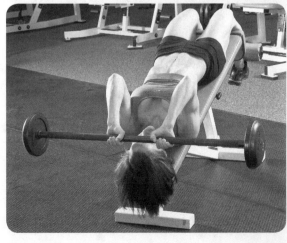

LYING BARBELL EXTENSION

Target	Triceps lateral and long heads
When	Early in workout
Start	Lie back on a flat bench while holding a barbell with a shoulder-width overhand grip. Begin with your arms extended toward the ceiling and the bar directly over your face.
Execution	While keeping your elbows in and your upper arms stationary, bend your arms to lower the bar to your forehead. Just before it touches, contract your triceps to extend your arms back to the start position.
Variations	Use an EZ-bar instead of a straight bar if it feels more comfortable. To target the triceps medial head, use a reverse grip (again, an EZ-bar might be more comfortable), which will likely require a lighter weight.
Advanced Tip	To further emphasize the long head, move your elbows back so your upper arms are at a 45-degree angle to the floor throughout; at the bottom of each rep, touch the bar to the top of your head.
Substitutes	Lying dumbbell extension, decline lying barbell extension, lying cable extension

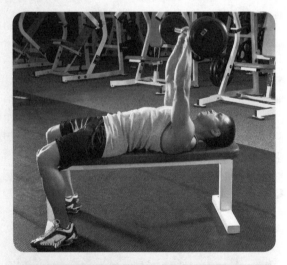

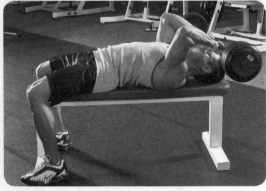

LYING DUMBBELL EXTENSION

Target   Triceps lateral and long heads

When   Early in workout

Start   Lie back on a flat bench while holding a pair of dumbbells. Begin with your arms extended toward the ceiling, the dumbbells over your face, and your palms facing each other.

Execution   Keeping your elbows in and your upper arms stationary, lower the dumbbells toward the sides of your head. When your hands are near forehead level, extend your elbows to return to the start position.

Variation   Begin with your palms facing forward at the top, then rotate your wrists to neutral by the end of each rep. Reverse the motion when going up.

Advanced Tip As with the barbell version, perform the exercise with your upper arms fixed at a 45-degree angle to the floor.

Substitutes Lying barbell extension, decline lying extension (dumbbell variation), lying cable extension

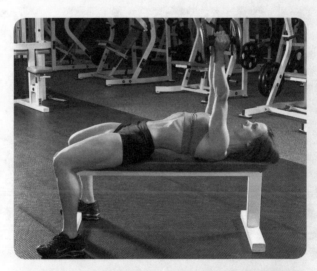

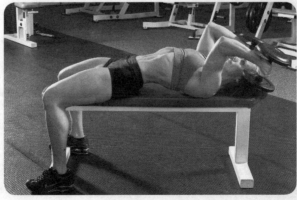

LYING CABLE EXTENSION

Target Triceps lateral and long heads

When Early to middle of workout

Start Attach a straight bar to a low pulley cable and place one end of a flat bench a foot or so (about 30 cm) away. Lie back on the bench with your head toward the cable, grasp the bar with a shoulder-width overhand grip, and begin with your arms extended toward the ceiling and the bar directly over your face.

Execution Bend your elbows to lower the bar to your forehead. When it touches, extend your elbows to press the bar back to the start position.

Variations Perform this exercise with an EZ-bar attachment or one arm at a time, using a handle attachment.

Advanced Tip Slide a decline bench (rather than a flat bench) into the cable station.

Substitutes Lying barbell extension, lying dumbbell extension, decline lying barbell extension

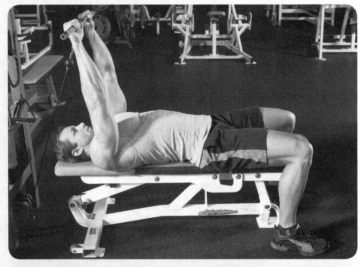

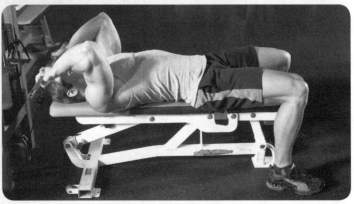

DIP—NARROW GRIP

Target	Triceps lateral and medial heads
When	Early in workout
Start	Find a dip apparatus with relatively narrow grips (no wider than shoulder width). Begin by holding on to the bars, with your body vertical and your arms extended.
Execution	Bend your arms to slowly lower yourself down, keeping your body vertical throughout. When your elbows reach roughly 90 degrees, press yourself back up to the start position.
Variations	Perform this movement on an assisted dip machine, which often allows you to adjust the grips to a narrower position. Another variation is to use a dip machine, in which you keep your back flat against the seat pad to keep your body vertical and maintain stress on the triceps, not the pectorals.
Advanced Tip	To increase resistance for fewer reps, do weighted dips by suspending a weight plate or dumbbell from a weight belt.
Substitute	Bench dip

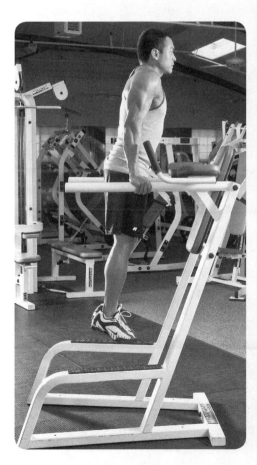
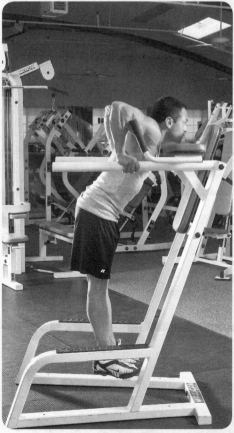

BENCH DIP

Target	Triceps lateral and medial heads
When	Middle to late in workout
Start	Position two flat benches a few feet apart and parallel with each other. Place your hands on one, with your arms extended and holding your body up just in front of the bench, and put the backs of your heels up on the other bench.
Execution	Bend your elbows to slowly lower your torso down toward the floor. When your upper arms reach parallel with the floor, extend your arms, keeping your elbows in, to press yourself back up to the start position.
Variation	For an easier version of the bench dip, place your feet on the floor in front of you, rather than on a bench.
Advanced Tip	For added resistance, place a weight plate (or multiple plates) on your lap before the set. (You may find it easier to have a partner place the weights on your lap for you.)
Substitute	Dip—narrow grip

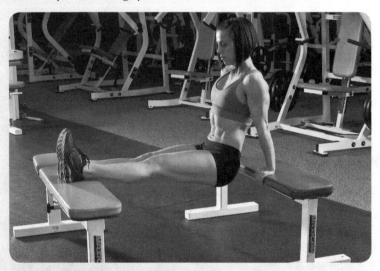

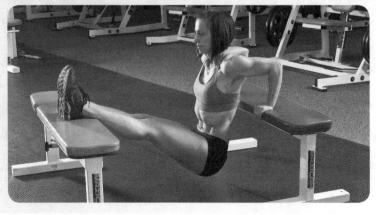

DUMBBELL OVERHEAD EXTENSION

Target	Triceps long head
When	Middle to late in workout
Start	Sit on a low-back seat while holding a relatively heavy dumbbell. Begin by holding the dumbbell overhead with both hands, palms against the upper inside plates, and thumbs and fingers overlapping.
Execution	Bend your elbows (without letting them flare out too much) to lower the dumbbell behind your head. When your elbows reach just past 90 degrees, extend your elbows to return to the start position.
Variations	Perform this exercise one arm at a time with a dumbbell that's about half the weight of the two-arm version. Place your nonworking hand on your hip and continue to lower the dumbbell behind your head but toward your opposite shoulder.
Advanced Tip	Perform overhead extensions either while seated on a flat bench or while standing; both versions of this exercise require more balance and core strength.
Substitutes	Barbell overhead extension, Smith machine overhead extension, cable overhead extension, seated overhead cable extension

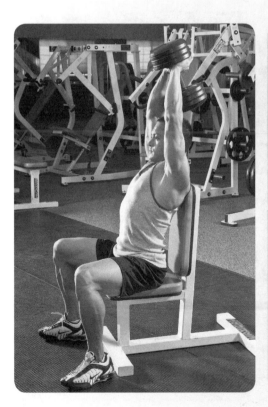 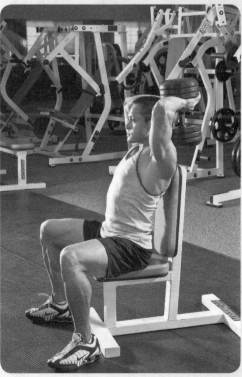

BARBELL OVERHEAD EXTENSION

Target   Triceps long head

When   Middle to late in workout

Start   Sit on a low-back seat while holding a barbell with an overhand grip no wider than shoulder width. Begin with the bar overhead and your arms extended.

Execution   Bend your elbows (without letting them flare out too much) to lower the bar behind your head. When your elbows reach just past 90 degrees, contract your triceps to extend your elbows and return to the start position.

Variations   Perform this exercise using an EZ-bar or on an incline bench, lowering the bar to the top of your head instead of behind it.

Advanced Tip To engage the core muscles to a greater extent, perform the movement while seated on an exercise ball.

Substitutes   Dumbbell overhead extension, Smith machine overhead extension, cable overhead extension, seated overhead cable extension

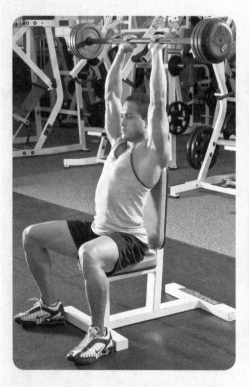 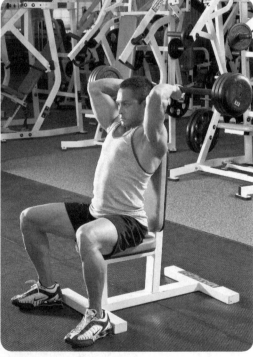

CABLE OVERHEAD EXTENSION

Target	Triceps long head
When	Middle to late in workout
Start	Attach a rope to a high pulley cable. Begin by facing away from the stack. Bend at the waist roughly 45 degrees, stagger your feet for balance, and hold the rope in both hands behind your head with your elbows bent.
Execution	Keeping your elbows in as much as possible, contract your triceps to extend your arms straight out in front of you. Hold the contraction for a count in the locked out position, then slowly return to the start position.
Variations	Use a straight bar or EZ-bar attachment in place of a rope.
Advanced Tip	At the top of each rep, turn your palms out and squeeze for extra contraction.
Substitutes	Seated overhead cable extension, dumbbell overhead extension, barbell overhead extension, Smith machine overhead extension

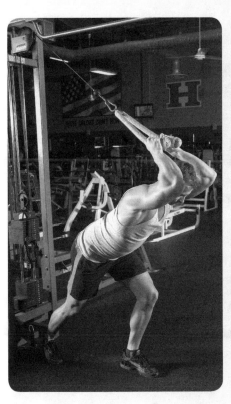 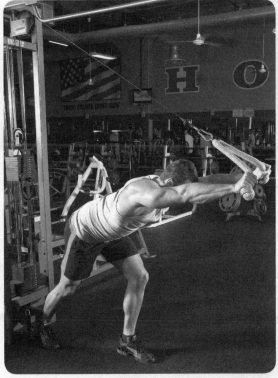

SEATED OVERHEAD CABLE EXTENSION

Target	Triceps long head
When	Middle to late in workout
Start	Position a low-back seat a foot or so (about 30 cm) in front of a cable stack, with a rope attached to the low pulley, or use a seated overhead cable extension machine (pictured). Face away from the cable stack. Grab the rope with both hands and begin while seated with your elbows bent, your hands behind your head, and your palms facing each other.
Execution	Keeping your elbows in as much as possible, contract your triceps to extend your arms overhead. Squeeze the contraction for a count with your elbows locked out, then return to the start position.
Variations	Perform the cable overhead extension with a straight bar or EZ-bar attachment (using an overhand grip), or do it one-handed by grabbing both ends of the rope with one hand.
Advanced Tip	At the top of each rep, turn your palms out and squeeze for a stronger contraction.
Substitutes	Dumbbell overhead extension, barbell overhead extension, Smith machine overhead extension, cable overhead extension

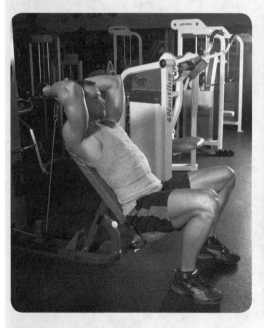 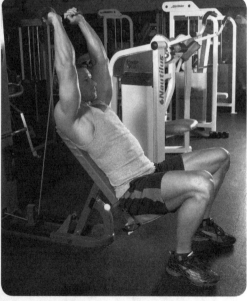

SMITH MACHINE OVERHEAD EXTENSION

Target	Triceps long head
When	Middle to late in workout
Start	Center a low-back seat in a Smith machine so that the bar is a foot or so (about 30 cm) behind the seat. Begin while seated, with the bar unhooked. Take a shoulder-width overhand grip, with your arms extended overhead (your hands will actually be behind your head).
Execution	While keeping your elbows in as much as possible, bend your arms to lower the bar down. When your arms reach 90 degrees, extend your elbows to return to the start position.
Variations	Do this exercise while seated on a flat bench or a high-back seat (an adjustable bench set one notch below vertical).
Advanced Tip	For a triceps superset, follow this exercise immediately with Smith machine close-grip bench presses.
Substitutes	Dumbbell overhead extension, barbell overhead extension, cable overhead extension, seated overhead cable extension

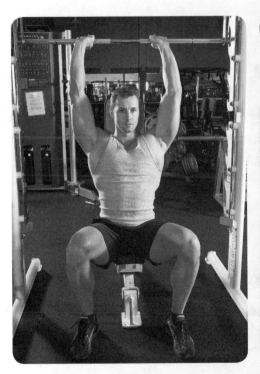 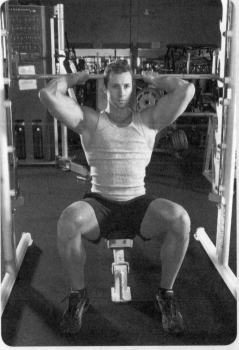

BARBELL BENCH PRESS—REVERSE GRIP

Target
Triceps medial head

When
Early in workout

Start
Lie back on a flat bench with a rack, and grasp a barbell with a shoulder-width reverse grip. Begin by holding the bar directly over your chest with your arms extended.

Execution
While keeping your elbows in, slowly lower the bar down to your lower pectorals. When it touches your chest, press the bar straight up to full elbow extension.

Variations
If a reverse grip aggravates your wrists, perform the exercise with a neutral-grip bar (if your gym has one). You can also perform reverse-grip bench presses in a Smith machine.

Advanced Tip
To deemphasize the bottom of the range of motion (where the pectorals, not the triceps, do most of the work), perform the exercise in a power rack and set the safety pins 6 to 12 inches (15 to 30 cm) above your chest so that the bar can't be lowered past that point.

Substitutes
Cable press-down—reverse grip, lying barbell extension (reverse grip)

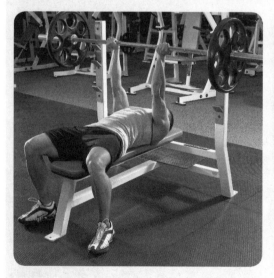
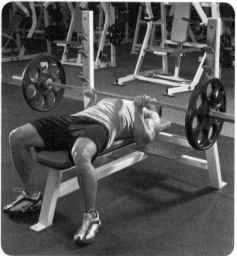

CABLE PRESS-DOWN–REVERSE GRIP

Target	Triceps medial head
When	Middle to late in workout
Start	Attach a straight bar to a high pulley cable. Stand facing the weight stack and grasp the bar with a shoulder-width, underhand grip. Begin with your forearms just above parallel with the floor and your elbows in close to your sides.
Execution	Keeping your elbows in, contract your triceps to extend your elbows until your arms are straight. Squeeze your triceps for a count, then return to the start position.
Variation	Perform this exercise one arm at a time by attaching a handle to the high pulley.
Advanced Tip	Use an EZ-bar attachment instead of a straight bar to turn the hands slightly inward and relieve pressure from the wrists.
Substitutes	Barbell bench press—reverse grip, lying barbell extension (reverse grip)

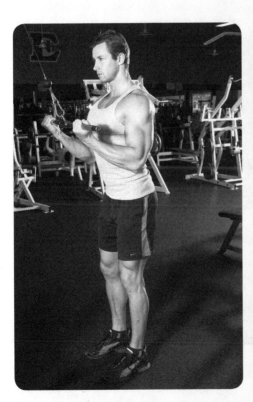 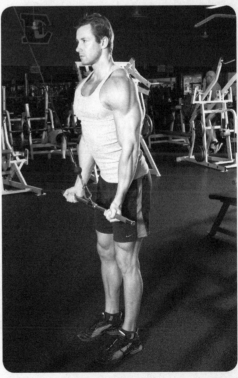

CHAPTER 8

Biceps and Forearm Exercises

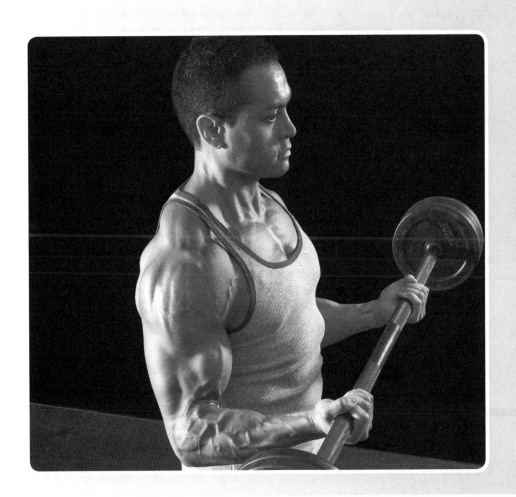

There's really only one major type of exercise for the biceps: the curl, in which the elbow is flexed against resistance. However, as you'll see in this chapter, there are many variations of the biceps curl that alter the position of the arms in relation to the rest of the body to train the muscles from various angles.

Because virtually all biceps exercises are single-joint movements—again, some variation of the curl—the rule on exercise order is to first do the exercises that allow you to lift the most weight in your workout (that is, barbell and dumbbell curls) followed by exercises such as preacher curls and concentration curls (wherein the upper arms are stabilized to promote further biceps isolation), which don't allow as much weight to be used. Curls that use cables and machines should typically be performed later in the workout as well.

Because the forearms are the smaller of the two muscle groups, they should be trained after the biceps (and typically in the same workout because of the proximity of the biceps and forearms and because the forearms assist on biceps exercises). The major exercises for below the elbow are reverse curls (similar to standard curls, only with a palms-down grip) and wrist curls. Hammer curls (in which the palms face each other) actually train both the biceps and the forearms and are a good bridge between biceps and forearm exercises.

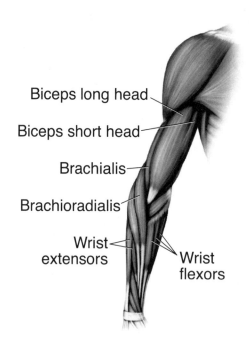

BARBELL CURL

Target	Biceps long and short heads
When	Early in workout
Start	Stand while holding a barbell with a shoulder-width grip and your arms extended down toward the floor. Keep your knees slightly bent.
Execution	While keeping your torso erect (don't lean back while lifting the weight), contract your biceps to curl the weight up. Make sure your elbows remain at your sides throughout—don't let them flare out or lift up. Slowly lower the weight to the start position.
Variations	Use either a straight bar or an EZ-curl bar on this exercise. Some people find the EZ-bar takes pressure off the wrists by putting them in a slightly more neutral position.
Advanced Tip	Take a closer grip (hip width or closer) to place more emphasis on the outer biceps head and a wider grip (greater than shoulder width) to place more emphasis on the inner head.
Substitutes	Cable curl, dumbbell curl

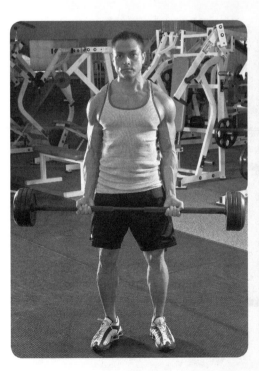 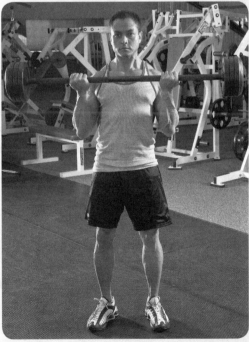

ALTERNATING DUMBBELL CURL

Target	Biceps long and short heads
When	Early in workout
Start	Stand while holding a pair of dumbbells at your sides with your arms extended toward the floor. Begin with your palms facing in and your knees slightly bent.
Execution	Keeping your elbow in at your side, curl one dumbbell up while simultaneously turning your palm up and out, so that at the top of the rep the palm faces slightly outward. Squeeze your biceps for a count in this position, then slowly lower the dumbbell back to the start position. Repeat with the other arm, and continue alternating arms.
Variations	Perform this exercise using both arms at a time or in a seated position.
Advanced Tip	Dumbbell curls lend themselves to a technique called running the rack (also known as drop sets): After reaching failure, immediately set the dumbbells down, grab a lighter pair, and rep out to failure with them. Continue down the rack until you're using extremely light dumbbells.
Substitutes	Incline dumbbell curl, concentration curl

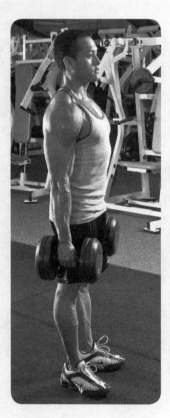 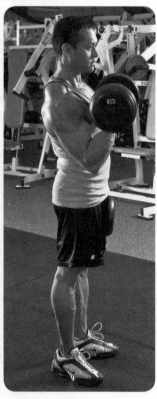

SEATED BARBELL CURL

Target   Biceps long and short heads

When   Early in workout

Start   Sit on a flat bench with a barbell on your lap and your feet flat on the floor. Grasp the bar with a shoulder-width grip, and begin with your arms bent roughly 90 degrees, your elbows in at your sides, and the bar on your upper thighs.

Execution   While keeping your upper body stationary (don't lean back) and your elbows in at your sides, curl the bar up as far as possible and squeeze your biceps. Lower the bar back to the start position, but do not let it rest completely on your legs between reps.

Variations Perform this exercise using an EZ-bar.

Advanced Tip Since the seated barbell curl accommodates only half the range of motion (to allow you to use more weight), you shouldn't use it in every biceps workout. A majority of your exercises should employ full movements with a full range of motion.

Substitutes Partial reps (top half of ROM) of barbell curl, dumbbell curl, cable curl

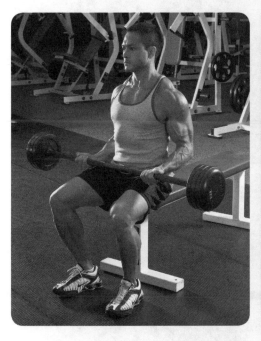 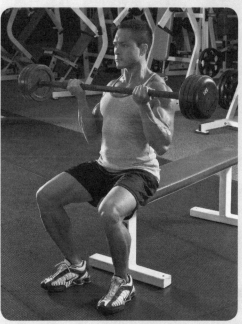

CABLE CURL

Target	Biceps long and short heads
When	Middle to late in workout
Start	Attach a straight bar to a low pulley cable. Stand a foot or two (30 to 60 cm) in front of the weight stack, and grasp the bar with a shoulder-width grip. Begin with your arms extended toward the floor and your knees slightly bent.
Execution	While keeping your elbows in at your sides, curl the weight up as far as possible. Squeeze the contraction for a count at the top, then return to the start position.
Variations	Use an EZ-bar attachment, or perform the exercise one arm at a time with a handle.
Advanced Tip	At the top of each rep, lift your elbows a few inches as you squeeze your biceps muscles to accentuate the contraction.
Substitutes	Barbell curl, dumbbell curl

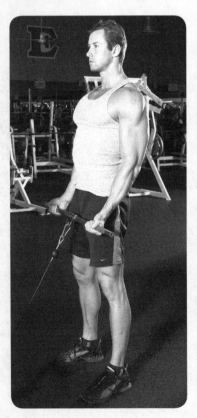 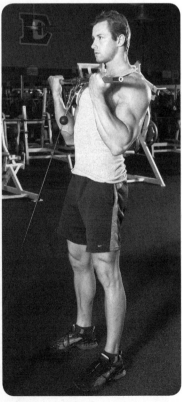

DRAG CURL

Target	Biceps long and short heads
When	Middle to late in workout
Start	Stand while holding a barbell in front of your thighs with your arms extended toward the floor, just as you would when doing a standard barbell curl.
Execution	Pull the bar straight up your body as high as possible (don't let it arc out in front of you) by contracting your biceps to bend your elbows. The bar should end up somewhere around your lower chest. Squeeze your biceps for a count at the top, then slowly lower the bar back down your body to the start position.
Variations	Because the bar is pulled straight up the body, you can do drag curls on a Smith machine. You can also perform them with dumbbells, using the same technique.
Advanced Tip	Drag curls on a Smith machine are a great way to overload the biceps with negative reps. Set the bar at about chest height, and slowly lower the bar using a count of three to five seconds. Have a spotter help you lift the bar back to the top, and repeat for five to eight reps.
Substitutes	None

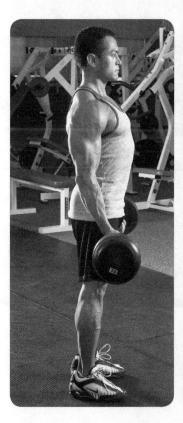 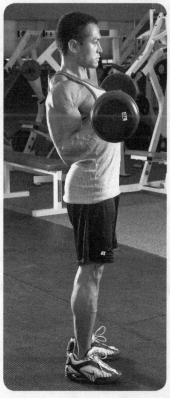

INCLINE CABLE CURL

Target	Biceps long and short heads
When	Middle to late in workout
Start	Position an incline bench equidistant between two cable stacks with handles attached to low pulleys. Grab the handles and lie back on the bench. Begin with your arms extended toward the pulleys and your palms facing the ceiling.
Execution	While keeping your upper arms stationary, simultaneously curl both handles toward you as far as possible. Squeeze your biceps hard for a count, then slowly return to the start position.
Variation	Do the movement one arm at a time, alternating arms every other rep.
Advanced Tip	If the cable apparatus allows, adjust the pulleys so that they're level with your shoulders, and perform the curl with your arms nearly parallel with the floor.
Substitutes	Incline dumbbell curl, cable curl, high cable curl

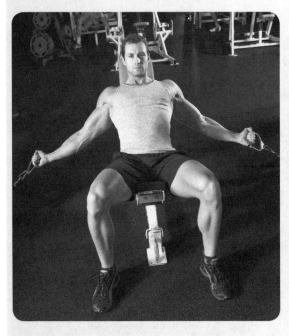 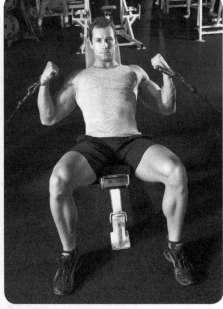

INCLINE DUMBBELL CURL

Target	Biceps long head
When	Middle to late in workout
Start	Lie back on an incline bench while holding a pair of dumbbells hanging straight toward the floor. Begin with your palms facing in.
Execution	Curl one dumbbell up, turning your palm up and out as you do so and keeping your elbow stationary. At the top of the rep, your palm should be facing slightly outward. Squeeze your biceps for a count, then slowly lower the dumbbell back down. Repeat with the other arm, alternating back and forth.
Variation	Perform reps using two arms at a time.
Advanced Tip	As you curl the weight up, let the dumbbell slide down your hand and settle against your fingers. This creates a longer lever arm for a stronger contraction.
Substitutes	Incline cable curl, dumbbell curl, concentration curl

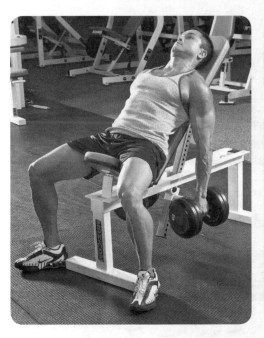 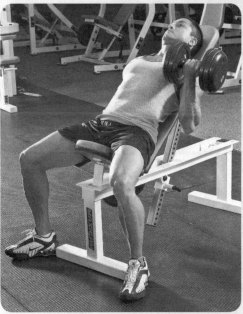

CONCENTRATION CURL

Target	Biceps long head
When	Late in workout
Start	Sit on a flat bench or seat with your feet flat on the floor in front of you. Hold a dumbbell in one hand, and keep your other hand on your leg for support. Begin bent over at the waist, with your working arm fully extended and hanging down between your legs and your elbow against your inner thigh.
Execution	While keeping your elbow against your leg to stabilize your upper arm, curl the weight up as far as possible, with your palm facing up throughout. Squeeze your biceps for a count at the top while turning your wrist out slightly, then return to the start position. Do all reps with that arm, then switch arms.
Variation	You can also do concentration curls while on your feet (bent over at the waist); hold on to a stable structure with your nonworking arm or place it on your leg.
Advanced Tip	To involve the biceps long head (which creates the biceps peak) even more as well as the brachioradialis (forearm) muscles, don't turn your palm up as you curl the weight; keep it facing in, as you would when doing hammer curls.
Substitutes	Cable concentration curl, lying cable concentration curl

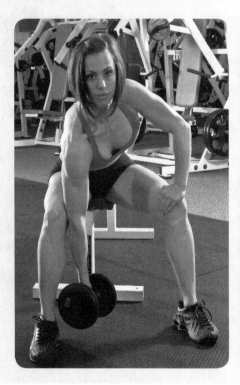 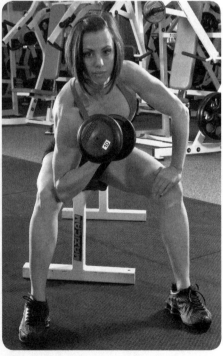

CABLE CONCENTRATION CURL

Target	Biceps long head
When	Late in workout
Start	Attach a handle to a low pulley cable. While standing a couple feet (about 60 cm) in front of the stack, hold the handle in one hand, bend over at your waist, and stabilize yourself by placing your non-working hand on your thigh or knee. Begin with your feet spread a couple feet apart, your working arm extended between your legs, your knees bent, and your elbow against your inner thigh.
Execution	While keeping your elbow in contact with your leg and the rest of your body still, curl the handle up as far as possible, with your palm facing up. At the top, squeeze the contraction for a count, then slowly lower to the start position. Do all reps with that arm, then switch arms.
Variation	Perform this exercise while seated on a bench or seat placed a couple feet in front of the stack.
Advanced Tip	Perform drop sets by simply moving the pin up the stack after reaching failure on a set.
Substitutes	Concentration curl, lying cable concentration curl

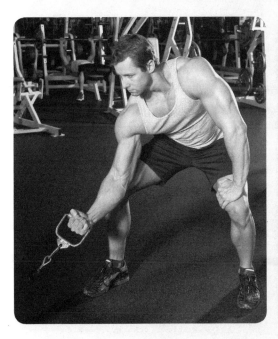 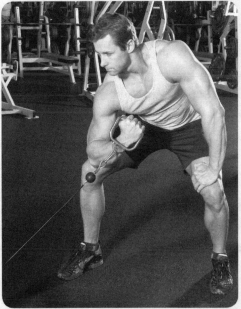

LYING CABLE CONCENTRATION CURL

Target	Biceps short head
When	Late in workout
Start	Attach a straight bar to a pulley set approximately halfway up the column (or to the high pulley if the cable apparatus doesn't adjust). Lie faceup on the floor or a bench, with your head a foot or so (about 30 cm) away from the stack, your knees bent, and your feet flat on the floor. Begin by holding the bar with a shoulder-width grip and your arms extended straight up.
Execution	While keeping your upper arms stationary, curl the bar to your forehead. Squeeze your biceps for a count when the bar reaches your head, then slowly return it to the start position.
Variations	Perform this exercise with an EZ-bar or rope attachment, or do one arm at a time using a handle.
Advanced Tip	Using the rope attachment, begin with your palms facing each other. As you curl the weight, rotate your wrists inward so that by the end of the rep your palms face slightly out.
Substitutes	Concentration curl, cable concentration curl

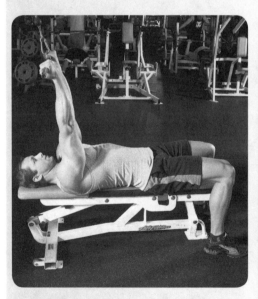 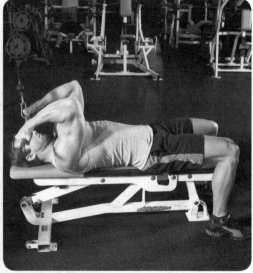

BARBELL PREACHER CURL

Target	Biceps short head
When	Middle to late in workout
Start	Sit on the seat of a preacher curl bench, and grasp a straight barbell with a shoulder-width grip. Begin with the backs of your upper arms flat against the pad and your elbows just short of fully extended.
Execution	While keeping your upper arms against the pad, curl the bar up as far as possible. Squeeze your biceps for a count at the top, then slowly lower the bar to the start position.
Variation	Use an EZ-bar to perform this exercise.
Advanced Tip	Instead of sitting on the seat, stand on the other side of the bench using the opposite side of the pad to stabilize your arms—this is often referred to as a Scott curl. Since that side of the pad is vertical (not angled), your upper arms will be hanging straight down toward the floor.
Substitutes	Dumbbell preacher curl, cable preacher curl, machine preacher curl

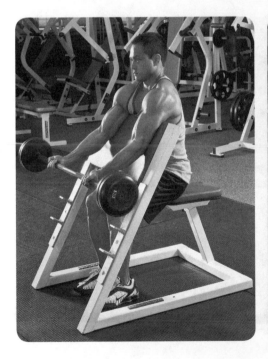 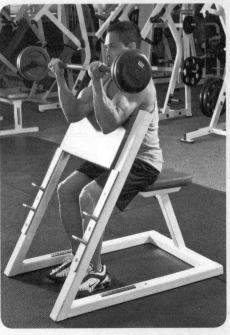

DUMBBELL PREACHER CURL

Target	Biceps short head
When	Middle to late in workout
Start	Sit on the seat of a preacher curl bench, and hold a dumbbell in one hand; use the other hand to hold on to the pad to stabilize yourself. Begin with the back of your upper arm (the working arm) flat against the pad and your elbow bent.
Execution	Extend your working elbow to slowly lower the dumbbell down. Just before reaching full elbow extension, curl the weight up, keeping your upper arm flat against the pad throughout. Squeeze the contraction for a count at the top. Do all reps with that arm, then switch arms.
Variation	Perform this exercise both arms at a time, holding a dumbbell in each hand.
Advanced Tip	For forced reps, use your nonworking hand to assist in lifting the dumbbell up.
Substitutes	Barbell preacher curl, cable preacher curl, machine preacher curl

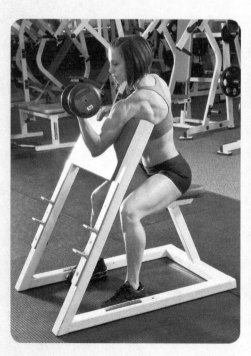 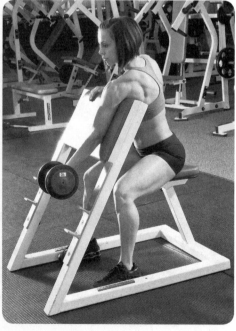

CABLE PREACHER CURL

Target	Biceps short head
When	Middle to late in workout
Start	Use a cable preacher curl machine (pictured), or position a preacher curl bench a couple feet (about 60 cm) in front of a cable stack with a straight-bar attachment on the low pulley. Grasp the bar with a shoulder-width grip, and sit down on the bench. Begin with your elbows extended but not locked out and the backs of your upper arms flat against the pad.
Execution	While keeping your upper arms against the pad, curl the weight up as far as possible. Squeeze the contraction for a count at the top, then slowly lower the bar to the start position.
Variations	Perform this exercise with an EZ-bar attachment, or curl one arm at a time using a handle attachment.
Advanced Tip	After reaching failure, finish the set by doing partial reps in only the top half of the range of motion.
Substitutes	Barbell preacher curl, dumbbell preacher curl, machine preacher curl

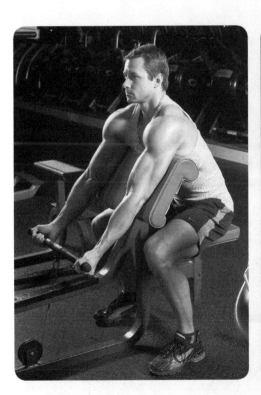 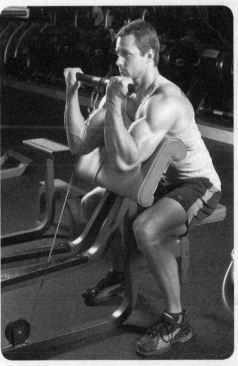

MACHINE PREACHER CURL

Target	Biceps short head
When	Middle to late in workout
Start	Adjust the seat of a preacher curl machine so that when you are in position your elbows line up with the machine's axis of rotation. Begin while seated and holding on to the bar, with your arms slightly bent and the backs of your upper arms flat against the pad.
Execution	Curl the bar up as far as possible, keeping your upper arms against the pad all the way up. Squeeze your biceps for a count, then return to the start position.
Variations	Several models of preacher curl machines exist, including the Hammer Strength brand (pictured). All essentially perform the same function.
Advanced Tip	Perform the movement one arm at a time with a machine that's properly balanced. You can either alternate arms every rep or do all reps with one arm and then switch arms.
Substitutes	Barbell preacher curl, dumbbell preacher curl, cable preacher curl

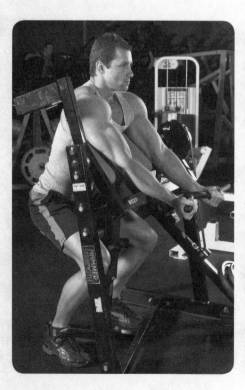 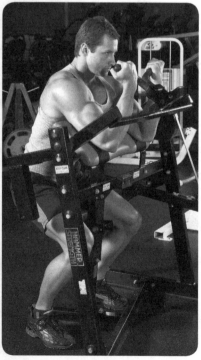

HIGH CABLE CURL

Target	Biceps short head
When	Late in workout
Start	Attach handles to high pulleys on either side of a cable crossover station. Stand directly in the middle of the station, grab the handles, and begin with your arms extended out to the sides so that your body forms a T.
Execution	While keeping your body and upper arms still, bend both elbows simultaneously to curl the handles in toward your head as far as possible. Squeeze the contraction for a count at the top, then return to the start position.
Variations	Alternate arms every rep to focus on each arm individually; or hold only one handle, and do all reps with that arm, then switch arms.
Advanced Tip	For a stronger contraction, at the top of each rep turn your palms so that they face behind you, and squeeze.
Substitutes	Cable curl, cable concentration curl

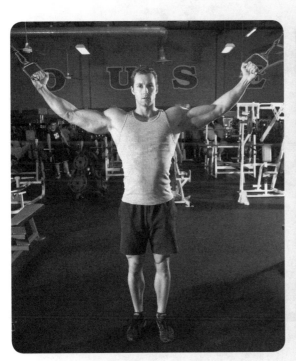 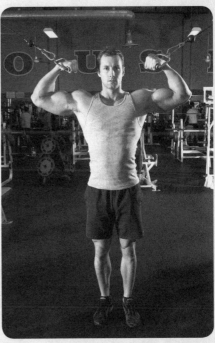

HAMMER CURL

Target	Biceps long head and brachialis
When	Late in workout
Start	Stand while holding a pair of dumbbells at your sides, with your palms facing in. Bend your knees slightly.
Execution	While keeping your elbows in at your sides and your upper arms stationary, curl the dumbbells up without rotating your wrists—keep your palms facing each other throughout. Squeeze the contraction for a count at the top, then return to the start position.
Variations	Perform hammer curls one arm at a time, in alternating fashion, or while seated.
Advanced Tip	To isolate the biceps and brachialis even further, perform hammer curls on a preacher bench. Do all reps with one arm, then switch arms.
Substitutes	Cable hammer curl

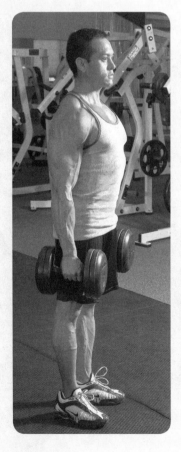 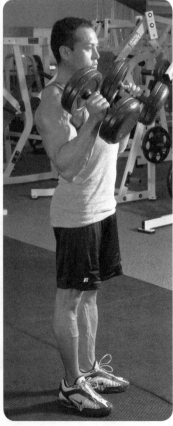

CABLE HAMMER CURL

Target	Biceps long head and brachialis
When	Late in workout
Start	Attach a rope to a low pulley cable. Stand while facing the stack and hold the rope with your palms facing each other and your thumbs up against the rubber stoppers. Begin with your arms extended toward the floor and your hands in front of your thighs.
Execution	While keeping your elbows in and your upper arms stationary, curl the rope up as far as possible without rotating your wrists. Squeeze the contraction for a count, then return to the start position.
Variation	Perform this exercise one arm at a time by holding both ends of the rope in one hand.
Advanced Tip	The weight stack makes it easy to do drop sets. After reaching failure, lighten the weight, by simply moving the pin up, and continue to rep out to failure.
Substitutes	Hammer curl

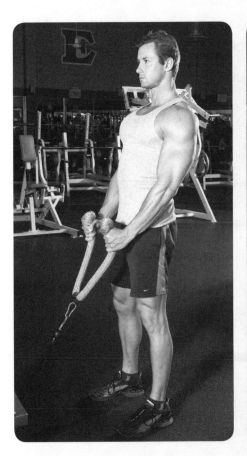
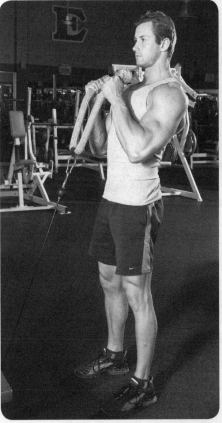

BARBELL REVERSE CURL

Target   Brachialis and brachioradialis

When   Late in workout

Start   Stand while holding a straight bar with an overhand grip and your knees slightly bent. Begin with your arms extended toward the floor and your hands in front of your thighs.

Execution   While keeping your elbows in at your sides and your upper arms stationary, curl the weight up as far as possible. Hold the contraction for a count, then slowly lower the bar to the start position.

Variation   Perform reverse curls with an EZ-bar, which may be easier on the wrists.

Advanced Tip   To place more emphasis on the brachioradialis, perform reverse curls with an open grip, keeping your thumb on top of the bar. This will force you to keep the bar closer to your body (as in a drag curl), causing more involvement of the brachioradialis.

Substitutes   Dumbbell reverse curl, cable reverse curl, preacher reverse curl

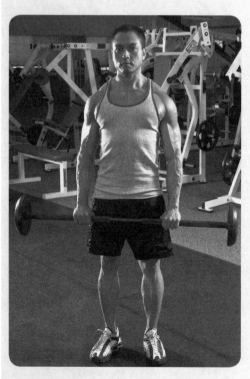 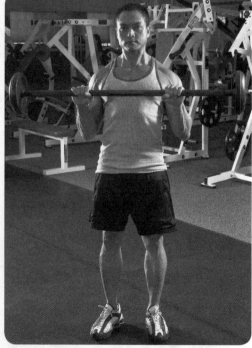

DUMBBELL REVERSE CURL

Target	Brachialis and brachioradialis
When	Late in workout
Start	Stand while holding a pair of dumbbells in front of your thighs, with your knees slightly bent.
Execution	While keeping your elbows in tight, your upper arms stationary, and your wrists in the reverse position, curl the dumbbells up as far as possible. Hold the contraction for a count, then slowly lower the dumbbells to the start position.
Variations	Perform this exercise one arm at a time in alternating fashion.
Advanced Tip	To involve the brachialis more, as you curl the weights up turn your wrists inward so that by the top of each rep your palms face each other, as with hammer curls.
Substitutes	Barbell reverse curl, cable reverse curl, preacher reverse curl

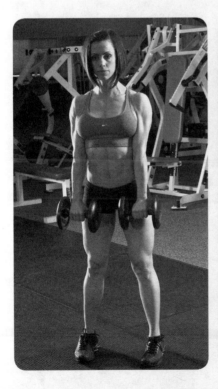 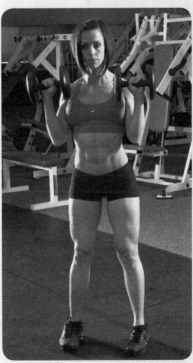

CABLE REVERSE CURL

Target	Brachialis and brachioradialis
When	Late in workout
Start	Attach a straight bar to a low pulley cable. Stand while facing the stack, and begin with a shoulder-width reverse grip (palms facing rearward), your arms extended toward the floor, and your knees slightly bent.
Execution	While keeping your elbows in at your sides and your upper arms stationary, curl the bar up as far as possible. Hold the contraction for a count, then return to the start position.
Variation	Perform this exercise with an EZ-bar attachment, which may relieve stress on the wrists.
Advanced Tip	To increase intensity, perform two or three drop sets after reaching failure with your initial weight.
Substitutes	Barbell reverse curl, dumbbell reverse curl, preacher reverse curl

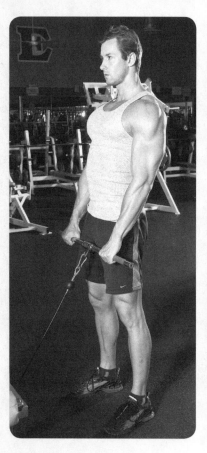
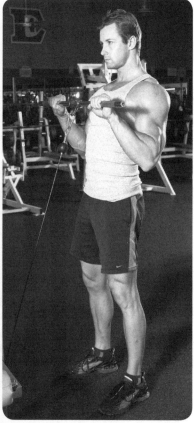

PREACHER REVERSE CURL

Target	Brachialis and brachioradialis
When	Late in workout
Start	Sit on a preacher bench, and grasp a straight barbell with a shoulder-width reverse grip. Begin with your arms extended and flush with the pad.
Execution	While keeping the backs of your upper arms in contact with the pad, curl the bar up as far as possible. Hold the contraction for a count, then slowly return the bar to the start position.
Variations	Perform this exercise with an EZ-bar, or do it one arm at a time with dumbbells.
Advanced Tip	Most people use a barbell shorter than an Olympic bar when doing preacher reverse curls. However, using a longer bar requires more balance and makes the exercise slightly more difficult, and it also improves grip strength.
Substitutes	Barbell reverse curl, dumbbell reverse curl, cable reverse curl

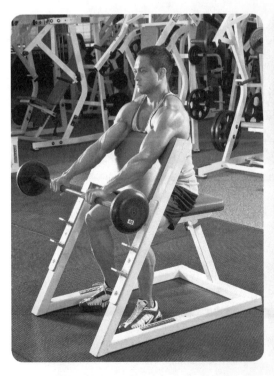
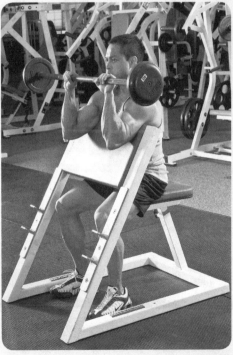

STANDING WRIST CURL

Target	Wrist flexors
When	After training biceps
Start	Stand while holding a straight barbell in front of your thighs with an underhand grip (palms facing forward), your arms extended toward the floor, and your wrists flat. Use an open grip, with your thumbs on the same side of the bar as your fingers.
Execution	While keeping both arms completely stationary, flex your wrists to lift the bar up in a short range of motion (only a few inches) so that at the top your palms face the ceiling. Squeeze the contraction for a count, then lower the bar to the start position.
Variations	Perform wrist curls with dumbbells, either lifting both simultaneously or alternating one at a time.
Advanced Tip	At the bottom of each rep, let the bar roll down your hands so that it settles in your fingers. This will provide a slightly greater stretch in the forearms.
Substitutes	Seated wrist curl, behind-the-back wrist curl

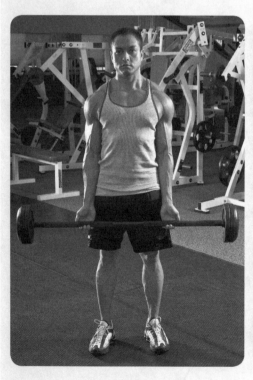 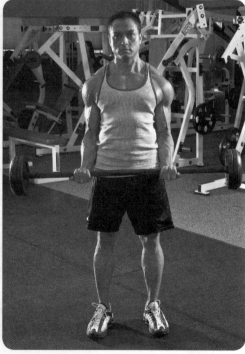

SEATED WRIST CURL

Target   Wrist flexors

When   After training biceps

Start   Sit in the middle of a flat bench with your legs straddling the bench. Hold a barbell with your hands about 6 inches (15 cm) apart, palms facing up. Bend over at the waist, and place the backs of your forearms against the bench, with your hands and wrists over the edge. Begin with your wrists extended so that your hands are below your forearms. Use an open grip (your thumbs on the same side of the bar as your fingers).

Execution   While keeping your arms stationary (as well as the rest of your body), flex your wrists as far as possible to lift the bar up and toward your upper arms in a short range of motion. Squeeze your forearms for a count, then return to the start position.

Variations   Use dumbbells, either lifting both simultaneously or one at a time.

Advanced Tip As with standing wrist curls, let the bar settle into your fingers at the bottom of each rep for a greater stretch.

Substitutes   Standing wrist curl, behind-the-back wrist curl

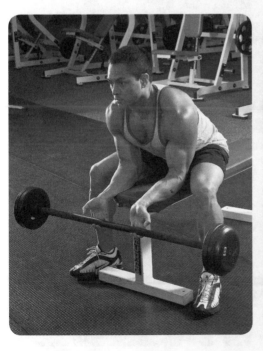 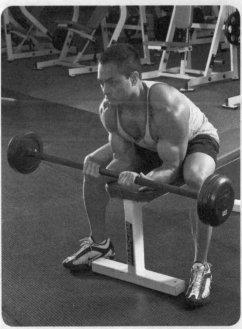

BEHIND-THE-BACK WRIST CURL

Target   Wrist flexors

When   After training biceps

Start   Stand while holding a barbell behind you with a shoulder-width grip
(palms facing back) and your arms extended toward the floor and
your wrists flat. Use an open grip (your thumbs on the same side of
the bar as your fingers).

Execution   While keeping your arms stationary, flex your wrists to lift the bar
up in a short range of motion so that your palms face the ceiling at
the top of the rep. Squeeze your forearms for a count, then return to
the start position.

Variation   Perform this exercise using a Smith machine.

Advanced Tip After doing straight sets, perform one last set isometrically by holding
the up position for as long as possible. This will provide an intense
burnout at the end of the workout.

Substitutes Wrist curl, seated wrist curl

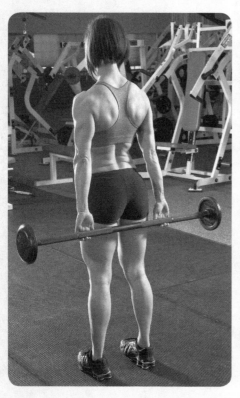
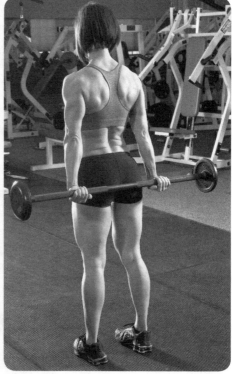

STANDING REVERSE WRIST CURL

Target	Wrist extensors
When	After training biceps
Start	Stand while holding a straight barbell in front of your thighs with an overhand grip (palms facing your thighs), your arms extended toward the floor, and your wrists flat.
Execution	While keeping both arms stationary, extend your wrists to lift the bar up in a short range of motion so that at the top your palms face the floor. Squeeze the contraction for a count, then lower the bar to the start position.
Variations	Perform reverse wrist curls with dumbbells or while seated on a flat bench as with seated wrist curls.
Advanced Tip	To exhaust both the posterior and anterior forearms in a short time, superset reverse wrist curls and regular wrist curls, performing both exercises to failure.
Substitutes	Barbell reverse curl, dumbbell reverse curl, preacher reverse curl, cable reverse curl

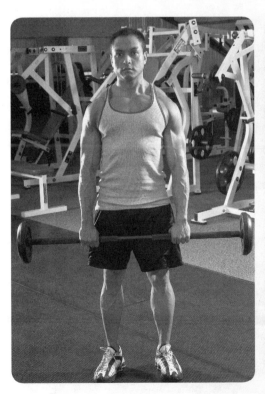 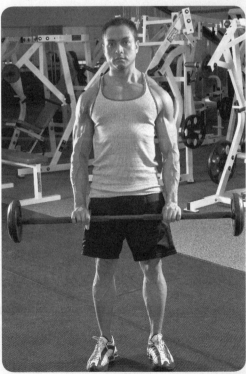

Rotator Cuff
Exercises

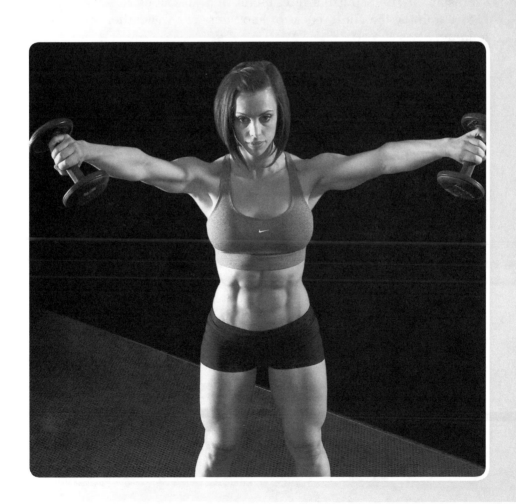

Training the muscles of the rotator cuff isn't about building them up to improve your physique aesthetically—at least not in the direct sense. Strengthening the rotator cuffs prevents injury so you can train at maximum intensity on all upper-body exercises, especially chest, shoulders, and back movements. The stress that training these muscle groups creates on the rotator cuff muscles is such that if the area is not properly conditioned to handle heavy loads, injury and possible surgery can occur, which could halt all lifting for many months. The bottom line is that a torn rotator cuff will negatively affect the rest of your training indefinitely. This chapter presents a collection of basic exercises to minimize such injuries and promote pain-free upper-body lifting.

Train the rotator cuff for 5 to 10 minutes two or three days per week. Select two or three of the exercises in this chapter and perform two or three sets of 15 to 20 reps. Always perform rotator cuff exercises at the end of a workout that involves other major muscle groups, because fatiguing the supraspinatus, infraspinatus, teres minor, and subscapularis (SITS) muscles before training the chest, back, or shoulders can make them susceptible to injury.

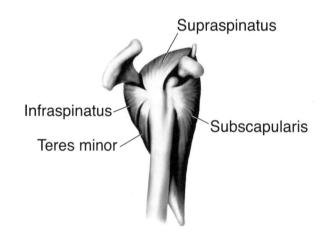

DUMBBELL EXTERNAL ROTATION

Target	Infraspinatus and teres minor
When	End of workout involving other major muscle groups
Start	Lie on your side on the floor or a flat bench while holding a very light dumbbell (5 to 10 pounds) in the hand of your upside arm (your opposite arm can remain on the floor or bench). Begin with your working arm bent 90 degrees, your elbow in tight at your side, and your forearm perpendicular to the floor and across your abdomen.
Execution	While keeping your arm bent and your elbow at your side, slowly pull the dumbbell up toward the ceiling until your forearm is roughly perpendicular to the floor. Slowly return to the start position. Complete all reps with that arm, then switch arms by turning over to the other side.
Substitute	Cable or elastic band external rotation

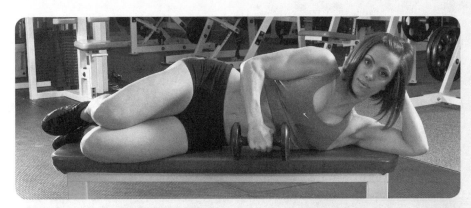

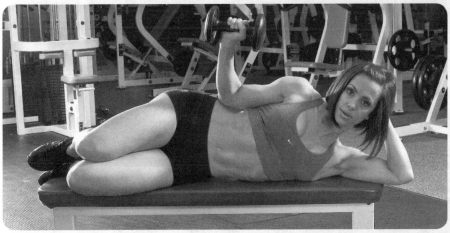

THREE-WAY RAISE

Target   Supraspinatus, infraspinatus, and teres minor

When   End of workout involving other major muscle groups

Start   Lie facedown on an incline bench set to approximately 30 degrees while holding a pair of light dumbbells. Begin with your arms hanging straight down toward the floor *(a)*.

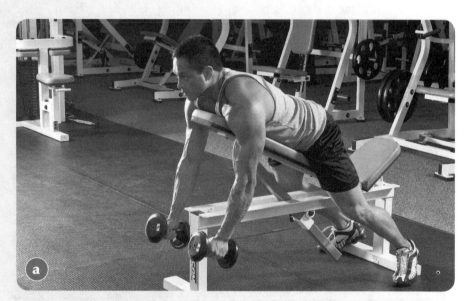

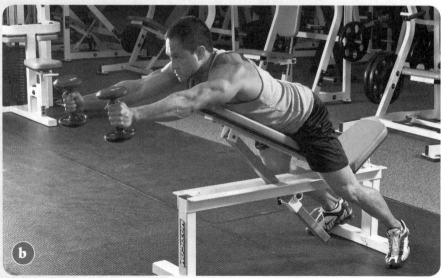

THREE-WAY RAISE (continued)

Execution   While keeping your arms extended, raise the dumbbells straight out in front of you until your arms are parallel with the floor *(b)*. Slowly lower the weights to the start position. Raise the dumbbells up and out to the sides until your arms are parallel with the floor *(c)*, then return to the start position. Raise the dumbbells up and back until your arms are parallel with the floor and in close to your sides *(d)*, then return to the start position once again. That's one repetition.

Substitute   Empty can

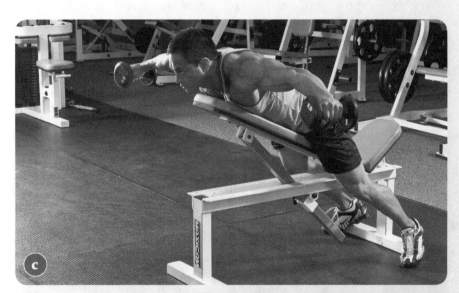

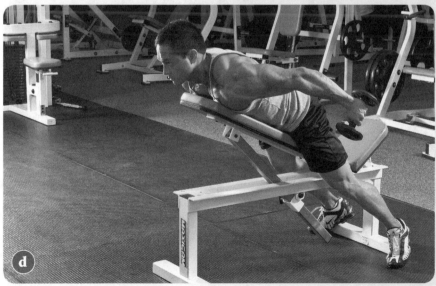

CABLE OR ELASTIC BAND EXTERNAL ROTATION

Target	Infraspinatus and teres minor
When	End of workout involving other major muscle groups
Start	Position a cable or elastic band with a handle at waist height (keep the resistance extremely light). Step away from the point of origin of the cable or band until you feel tension. While facing sideways, begin by holding the handle in the hand farther away from the point of origin, with that forearm across your body and the elbow in tight to your side.
Execution	While keeping your arm bent and your elbow in at your side, slowly pull the handle out and back until your forearm is roughly perpendicular to your abdomen. Slowly return to the start position. Complete all reps with that arm, then switch arms, facing the opposite direction.
Substitute	Dumbbell external rotation

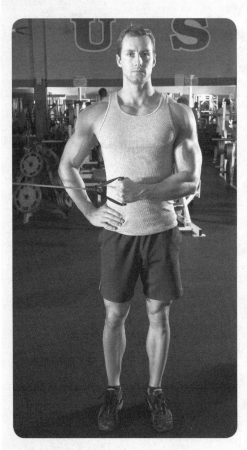
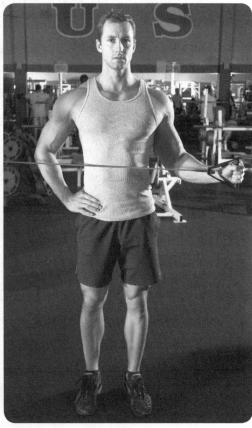

DUMBBELL INTERNAL ROTATION

Target
Subscapularis

When
End of workout involving other major muscle groups

Start
Lie on your side on a flat bench while holding a very light dumbbell (5 to 10 pounds) in the hand of your downside arm (keep the upside arm rested along your side). Begin with your working arm bent 90 degrees, with your elbow in tight at your side and your forearm parallel with the floor.

Execution
While keeping your arm bent and your elbows at your side, slowly pull the dumbbell up until your forearm touches your midsection. Slowly return to the start position. Complete all reps with that arm, then switch arms by turning over to the other side.

Substitute
Cable or elastic band internal rotation

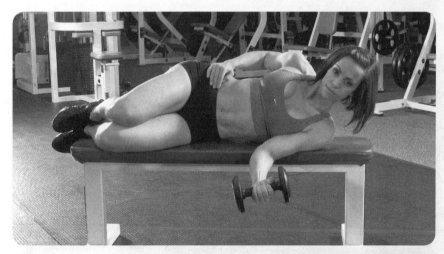

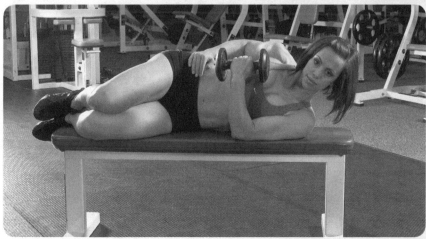

CABLE OR ELASTIC BAND INTERNAL ROTATION

Target   Subscapularis

When   End of workout involving other major muscle groups

Start   Position a cable or elastic band with a handle at waist height (keep the resistance extremely light). Step away from the point of origin of the cable or band until you feel tension. While facing sideways, begin by holding the handle in the hand closer to the point of origin, with that forearm perpendicular to your torso, your arm bent 90 degrees, and your elbow in tight to your side.

Execution   While keeping your arm bent and your elbow in at your side, slowly pull the handle toward you until your forearm reaches your midsection. Slowly return to the start position. Complete all reps with that arm, then switch arms, facing the opposite direction.

Substitute Dumbbell internal rotation

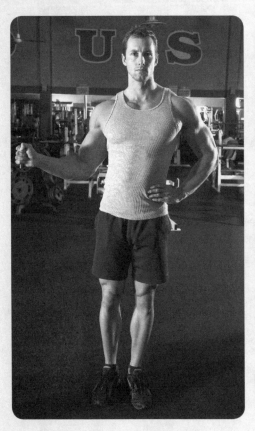 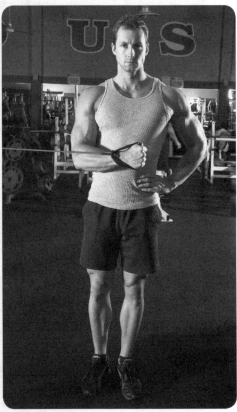

EMPTY CAN

Target	Supraspinatus
When	End of workout involving other major muscle groups
Start	Stand while holding a pair of light dumbbells at arms' length in front of your thighs.
Execution	With your thumbs pointed downward and while keeping your arms straight, slowly lift the dumbbells (creating a V shape with your arms) until your arms reach just past parallel with the floor. Pause for a count, then slowly return to the start position.
Substitute	Three-way raise

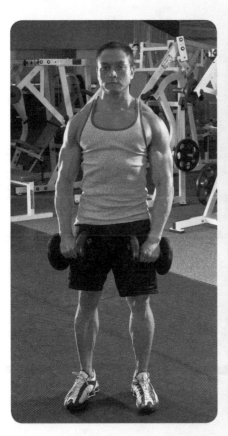
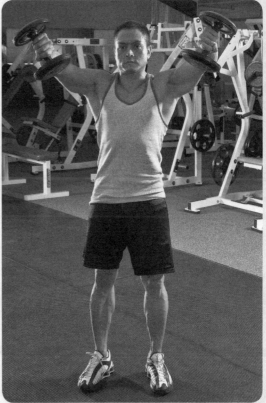

PART III

Advanced Applications

CHAPTER 10

Advanced
Training Methods

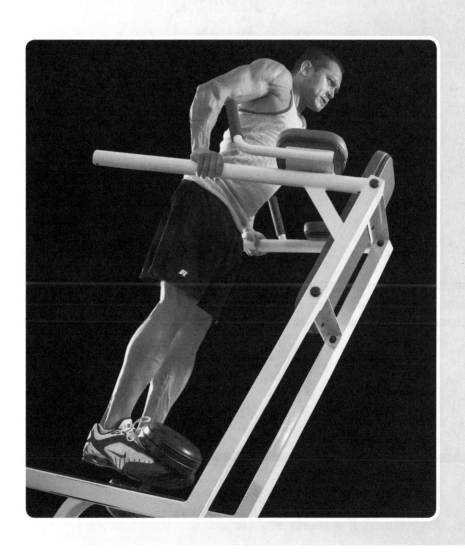

For beginning or intermediate lifters, sticking to basic training principles might be the best approach because the muscles likely have yet to adapt to even the most rudimentary lifting methods. But after a time—whether it be six months, a year, or even two years—your body will require more aggressive modes of training in order for you to continue to see increases in muscular size, strength, and endurance.

Increasing intensity is the key, and the longer you've trained, the more creative and innovative you'll need to be to make your workouts more intense. Hence, many of the following advanced training techniques are specifically recommended as a means of boosting intensity, whereas others provide a new stimulus to promote continuing results.

SUPERSETS

As the most widely used of all intensity-boosting techniques, a superset involves doing two different exercises back to back without resting. Virtually any two exercises can be paired for a superset. For example, to work the chest you can do a set of flat bench dumbbell presses and then proceed immediately to a set of dumbbell flys, resting only as long as it takes you to transfer from the first to the second exercise. Another example of a superset for one muscle group is overhead presses followed by lateral raises for the shoulders. Typically, you'd do three or four supersets in this fashion, resting between each superset.

The previous examples involve two exercises for the same muscle group. This is a very common practice as a means of exhausting a single muscle group to promote the muscle fiber breakdown that can lead to muscle growth. In both examples, notice how a compound exercise precedes an isolation move. Because the muscles will be more fatigued while doing the second exercise, it makes sense to do the compound move first so that you can maximize the amount of weight used. However, there's nothing wrong with pairing two compound exercises or even two isolation exercises. We simply suggest doing the exercise that allows you to lift more weight first. That said, you can also do the isolation exercise first, followed by the compound move, to combine supersets with the high-intensity technique known as preexhaustion (see page 194 in this chapter) for twice the intensity.

Pairing opposing muscle groups, such as the chest and back or the triceps and biceps, is also very common. A good example of a chest–back superset is a flat or incline bench dumbbell press followed by a rowing exercise (see table 10.1 for a chest–back superset routine). A triceps–biceps superset might consist of a cable press-down and a barbell curl. (More supersets can be found in chapters 11 and 12.) Research

TABLE 10.1 Chest–Back Superset Routine

Perform the pair of exercises in each superset back to back without resting. After each superset, rest 1 to 2 minutes and repeat each superset twice for a total of 3 supersets.

	Sets	Reps	Rest
SUPERSET 1	3		1-2 min between supersets
Incline dumbbell press		8-10	
Barbell bent-over row		8-10	
SUPERSET 2	3		1-2 min between supersets
Wide-grip pull-up		6-10	
Weighted dip		6-10	
SUPERSET 3	3		1-2 min between supersets
Cable crossover		12-15	
Straight-arm pull-down		12-15	

has suggested that, because a muscle tends to receive a strength boost immediately after an intense contraction of its antagonist (a muscle that performs the opposite movement), you might actually be stronger on the exercise performed second in the superset than when performing that exercise via straight sets. Thus when supersetting opposing muscle groups, alternate the muscle that goes first in the superset so that both muscles gain the benefit from being trained second.

Supersets can also train different but nonopposing muscle groups, such as the shoulders and triceps, the chest and biceps, and any number of other combinations. In these instances, the major benefit of supersetting is that you're essentially doing twice the sets in the same amount of time as when doing straight sets. You will save time by the end of the workout, provided you're doing the same number of sets as before. By minimizing rest periods, you'll also extend each bout of lifting, which will keep your heart rate elevated for longer periods. Whereas when doing a straight set you might be lifting for 30 to 45 seconds at a time, a superset typically involves a bout of lifting twice as long, keeping your heart rate up that much longer. This is why supersetting is often the lifting method of choice for those looking to add a cardiorespiratory element into their weight training for increased calorie burning and better overall conditioning.

Tri-Sets and Giant Sets

Supersetting can also involve more than two exercises. Three exercises performed consecutively without rest is called a tri-set; more than three is referred to as a giant set. All types of supersets speed up a workout, increase intensity by allowing limited rest between exercises, and maintain an elevated heart rate, but tri-sets and giant sets offer a means of training more than two muscle groups together or exhausting a single muscle even further. For example, you can use tri-sets to train the three different pushing muscles of the upper body: the chest, shoulders, and triceps. This might consist of flat or incline bench presses (either barbell or dumbbell) for the chest, followed by overhead presses to train the shoulders, and then either press-downs or lying extensions for the triceps. Another effective tri-set could include all pulling exercises: lat pull-downs or rows for the back, followed by upright rows or lateral raises for the shoulders, then curls for biceps.

Tri-sets are also effective for thoroughly working a muscle group with three different exercises. As with supersets, it's best to do the exercise that allows you to use the heaviest weight first and to do the move with the lightest weight last. For example, a chest tri-set might consist of barbell presses, dumbbell presses, and any type of fly exercise, in that order. For shoulders, you'd do overhead presses, upright rows, then lateral raises (see table 10.2); a back tri-set could be bent-over rows, lat pull-downs, then straight-arm pull-downs.

Giant sets are a further extension of tri-sets in which one muscle group can be trained with four or more exercises or four or more muscle groups can be trained one after the other. (Table 10.3 provides a sample upper-body giant set.) Doing four or more exercises consecutively for the same muscle group (rather than two or three exercises) is simply a means of adding even more intensity to a particular area. When performing giant sets, keep in mind that you're increasing overall volume on the given

TABLE 10.2   Shoulder Tri-Set

Perform the exercises in the following tri-set consecutively without resting. After each tri-set, rest 1 to 2 minutes. Complete 3 or 4 tri-sets.

	Sets	Reps
TRI-SET	3-4	
Dumbbell overhead press		8-10
Barbell upright row		10-12
Dumbbell lateral raise		12-15

TABLE 10.3 Upper-Body Giant Set

Perform the exercises in the following giant set consecutively, resting only as long as it takes to move to the next exercise. After each giant set, rest 1 to 2 minutes. Complete 3 giant sets.

	Sets	Reps
GIANT SET	3	
Flat bench dumbbell press		8-10
Seated cable row		8-10
Smith machine overhead press		8-10
Dumbbell curl		8-10
Lying triceps extension		8-10

muscle, and be wary of overtraining. Normally you might do nine total supersets for a single muscle group, but you should do only four or five giant sets because each giant set includes at least twice the volume of a single superset.

Extended Sets

An extended set is a subtle variation of a superset, tri-set, or giant set. But an extended set differs from the others in that it's basically the same movement performed two or more different ways by changing the angle of the exercise or the grip position or both. For example, doing an incline dumbbell press, flat bench dumbbell press, and a decline dumbbell press consecutively constitutes an extended set. Though all three are technically different exercises, they are essentially the same movement (in each, you press dumbbells straight up). All that changes from one to the other is the bench angle. An example of an extended set for back is a wide-grip lat pull-down; a close-grip pull-down; and a close, reverse-grip pull-down. All involve the same movement, each with a different grip.

The order in which you do the exercises in the extended set is crucial. In the aforementioned examples, notice how the toughest variation of the three (incline for the chest and wide-grip pull-down for the back) is done first, and the easiest (decline and reverse grip) last. Getting the most out of extended sets depends on increasing the body's mechanical advantage from set to set. In fact, that's the whole point of extended sets.

Changing to a more biomechanically advantageous angle of the exercise allows you to continue or extend the set. If you did exercises in the opposite order, from easiest to hardest, you'd be able to get more reps on decline presses and reverse-grip pull-downs, but by the time you got to incline and wide-grip pull-downs, you'd be too fatigued to perform an appreciable number of reps. In addition to boosting intensity, extended sets offer the benefit of targeting a variety of muscle fibers in a muscle in the course of just one set.

To perform an extended set, choose a weight for the first exercise that normally limits you to four or five reps (even though you will attempt no more than four reps). For each change in grip or angle in that extended set, you will attempt two to four reps. Don't do more than four reps on any exercise, except for the final exercise of an extended set, wherein you can rep out to failure. If you have three or four exercise changes per extended set, you will end up doing a total of about 7 to 16 reps. So in essence, you'll use a weight for each exercise that's best for strength gains, but at the end of the extended set the total reps that you've done for that muscle group fall in the range that is optimal for growth. Refer to table 10.4 for sample extended sets for the shoulders, triceps, and biceps.

TABLE 10.4 **Sample Extended Sets**

For each muscle group, do exercises consecutively (without rest) in the following order:

Shoulders
Dumbbell bent-over lateral raise
Dumbbell front raise
Dumbbell lateral raise
Triceps
Reverse-grip cable press-down
Cable press-down (overhand grip)
Biceps
Reverse-grip barbell curl
Barbell curl

DROP SETS

Descending sets (more commonly referred to as drop sets) provide a means of not only training to failure on a given set but also training past failure to boost intensity in a workout for potentially greater gains in muscular size, strength, and endurance. A drop set involves performing a set of a particular exercise to failure, then immediately decreasing the weight (resting only as long as it takes you to change the weight) and repping out to failure with the lighter weight on the same exercise. You can repeat this process, continuing to decrease weight until you've completed multiple drop sets. A typical routine involves doing one or two such sets on a specific exercise, doing two or three drop sets on each. Drop sets are a great technique for training past failure, but they should be used sparingly. Using this technique on more than one or two sets of an exercise for an extended period will lead to overtraining.

Drop sets tend to work best for an exercise that allows you to decrease weight quickly and conveniently. Any cable or machine exercise, regardless of what muscle group it's training, that uses a weight stack will lend itself to drop sets because it takes only a few seconds to move the pin up the stack to lighten the weight. Dumbbell exercises also work well. Running the rack is a means of drop-setting in which you might begin with 40-pound dumbbells for standing curls, rep out to failure, then decrease the weight in 5- to 10-pound increments, taking each drop set to failure, until you're using dumbbells as light as 10 to 15 pounds and your biceps are fully exhausted. See table 10.5 for another example of using dumbbells for drop sets.

TABLE 10.5 **Running the Rack With Shoulders**

Here's a sample progression of an effective series of drop sets for dumbbell lateral raises. Select a weight that will have you fail at 8 to 10 reps, then decrease the weight in 5-pound increments in each successive set.

Weight	Reps
35-pound dumbbells	8-10 (to failure)
30-pound dumbbells	to failure
25-pound dumbbells	to failure
20-pound dumbbells	to failure
15-pound dumbbells	to failure

You can perform drop sets on virtually any exercise that you'd like to add intensity to. For example, doing a drop set while doing bench presses or bent-over barbell rows is as easy as taking a 10- or 25-pound plate off each side of the bar to decrease weight. It's typically recommended that you decrease the weight by about 20 to 30 percent on each drop.

REST-PAUSE SETS

Like drop sets, rest-pauses allow you to train past the point of initial muscular failure. But instead of decreasing weight to continue, you rest 10 to 20 seconds and then rep out to failure with the same weight, albeit for fewer reps than you were able to perform initially. For example, to do rest-pause sets on Smith machine overhead presses, select a weight that you could do for about 6 reps. Complete 5 or 6 reps, then rest 10 to 20 seconds, do 2 or 3 more reps, and rest again. Then, do two or three more sequences of the 2 or 3 more reps and a rest to accomplish one rest-pause set. As a result, you're able to do a set of 11 to 15 reps (or more) with a weight that you can normally do for just 5 or 6 reps. This will increase training intensity and develop muscular strength.

You can use rest-pauses with most any exercise (see table 10.6 for a sample chest rest-pause set); but, as with drop sets, exercises in which you can easily set down or rack the weight tend to be more practical. Rest-pause sets are extremely taxing on muscles and joints and can quickly lead to overtraining, so don't overdo them—limit rest-pauses to the last one or two sets of an exercise, and don't do them regularly for more than a month or so.

TABLE 10.6   Sample Rest–Pause Set for Machine Chest Press

Weight	Reps	Rest
200 pounds	6	15 seconds
200 pounds	2-3	15 seconds
200 pounds	2-3	15 seconds
200 pounds	2-3	15 seconds

FORCED REPS

The premise with forced reps is also training past failure, but instead of decreasing weight after reaching failure (drop sets) or resting (rest-pause), you'll continue to do reps with the same weight with the help of a spotter. The objective, as with rest-pauses, is to do significantly more reps with a particular weight than your body is capable of with straight sets. For example, when doing a set of bench presses, you'd take the set to failure, at which point your spotter helps you just enough to be able to get two or three more challenging reps. The work of the spotter is crucial. If the spotter helps too much, you won't work hard enough to get the full benefit of forced reps. On the other hand, if the spotter doesn't help enough, you likely won't be able to get more reps. You can also do forced reps without a spotter on unilateral exercises by using the nonworking arm to assist, as well as on machines that have a foot plate that moves the handles (as some chest press machines have).

Forced reps are one of the most effective advanced techniques for increasing muscular strength and size. But at the same time, they put such a stress on the muscles and joints that overtraining is inevitable if you do them too frequently. As a rule, do not do forced reps in every workout; when doing them, limit them to only the last one or two sets of an exercise. And again, as with rest-pauses and drop sets, you can use forced reps on virtually any exercise.

PARTIAL REPS

You can perform reps through less than a full range of motion to achieve three distinct goals: Add intensity to a set by training past muscular failure; concentrate on a particularly weak portion of an exercise's ROM to increase overall strength in that lift, which can eventually lead to gains in size as well; and overload a muscle in the strongest part of its ROM to spark muscular growth.

When simply looking for a boost in intensity, perform partials after reaching failure on a set with full-ROM reps (as opposed to doing an entire set of partial reps). For example, when you do seated rows, the most difficult part of the ROM is the last portion, when your hands are closer to your midsection. Therefore, at the point in the set when you can no longer pull the handle to your midsection, do reps in only the first half of the ROM (the easier portion), from the point where your arms are fully extended to where the are partially bent. Do partials that way until you reach failure again and can no longer move the handle even a few inches. In general, the easiest portion of the ROM is the limited range at which you do partials.

When working on a weak point in an exercise's ROM, do the entire set using partials (do no full-ROM reps). For example, with biceps curls, the weak portion is the bottom half, from the arms-extended position to the point where your elbows are at 90 degrees. The entire set will be in this limited ROM. During any type of barbell, dumbbell, or machine press (for the chest or shoulders), the weak part of the ROM is the bottom half. If using a barbell, have a spotter present to help you rerack the bar if and when you reach failure.

To overload the strongest part of an exercise's ROM, first select a weight that's heavier than you'd normally use, since the weak portion won't be limiting your strength as usual. On most exercises you'll do the top half of the ROM, so a power rack or Smith machine with adjustable safety pins is most effective. The reason is that you need to make sure you don't lower the weight past the point at which the muscles are at their strongest; safety pins will ensure this. For example, to do partials on barbell presses (whether it be flat bench, incline, decline, or overhead presses), set the pins so that you'll begin each rep with your elbows at greater than 90 degrees. On each rep, that is your starting point, and you'll press up from there to an arms-extended position to complete the partial rep.

When doing partials to increase strength on the weaker ROM of an exercise or to overload the stronger ROM of a lift, perform the partials first in the workout (when you're at your strongest) and follow them immediately with full-ROM training for that exercise and muscle group. If you are doing partials as a means of extending a set past failure, don't do more than two sets on an exercise. More will lead to overtraining. You should also limit partials to one exercise for each muscle group in a given workout. If you prefer to do partial reps on more than one exercise, then do only one set of partials for each. Doing complete sets of partials too often can be problematic, even if you don't take the sets to failure. When the underused portion (which hasn't been trained through full ROM on a regular basis) is eventually called into play on other lifts or during athletic activities, it may be susceptible to injury.

SLOW-REP TRAINING

Chapter 3 discusses appropriate rep speed and notes that the concentric (positive) and eccentric (negative) portions each take a couple seconds or so to complete. But altering rep speed can sometimes be beneficial in your training, both to promote variety and to achieve specific goals.

Performing reps at a very slow pace maximizes muscle growth because of the principle of time under tension (see page 36 in chapter 3). In short, extending the duration of each rep (the period in which your muscles are under the tension of resistance) will increase the muscles' potential for growth.

One slow rep should take approximately 5 seconds on the positive and 5 seconds on the negative. For example, a set of 10 reps on preacher curls at a slow pace would take a little over 90 seconds to complete, which is more than twice as long as it would take to do 10 normal-speed reps. With normal-speed reps, you typically perform the positive faster than the negative; with slow reps, however, you should do both phases at the same speed. The weight you select for a set of slow reps will likely need to be lighter than that of a regular set, provided you're aiming for the same number of reps. You can perform slow reps on most exercises, though we recommend selecting those exercises that allow you to drop or rack the weight safely upon reaching failure (assuming you don't always have a spotter present), because this technique fatigues the muscles rather quickly.

Use slow-rep sets only occasionally in your training. Select just one or two exercises and do three or four sets of slow reps. Remember that normal-speed reps should make up the majority of your sets.

BALLISTIC TRAINING

Whereas slowing down rep speed can maximize growth, performing each rep in a set as fast and explosively as possible (ballistically) will develop strength and power by maximizing the recruitment of fast-twitch muscle fibers. You can also enhance muscle growth through ballistic training, albeit indirectly. The stronger you become, the more weight you'll be able to use in the future on a particular exercise for the same number of reps, which can lead to hypertrophy. In addition, fast-twitch fibers have more growth potential than slow-twitch fibers, which is another reason why using fast reps fosters hypertrophy.

With ballistic training, you do the negative portion of each rep under control instead of dropping the weight. On the positive portion, though, you press or pull the weight (depending on the exercise) as quickly as possible through a full ROM, often to the point that the weight leaves your hands because of the increased speed of the rep.

Exercise selection, amount of resistance, rep count, and even rest periods are crucial when doing ballistic reps. Not all exercises lend themselves to being performed explosively because safety becomes a more valid concern with this style of training. For example, free-weight pressing exercises for the chest, in which the bar or dumbbells are directly over you and could be dropped them if you lose control, aren't the best choices for ballistic training.

Machines, especially Smith machines, are often the ideal equipment, since the weight can safely leave your hands at the top of a rep. Because the path of motion is fixed, it will be much easier to catch the bar coming back down than it would be with free weights. Examples of appropriate exercises are Smith machine flat bench, incline, or decline press (chest); Smith machine one-arm row (back); and Smith machine overhead press and upright row (shoulders). For arms, cable curls (biceps) and press-downs (triceps) lend themselves to ballistic reps.

The amount of weight you use for explosive reps needs to be much lighter—approximately half the resistance—than you would use for normal-speed reps. The whole point of ballistic training is to move the weight on the concentric portion much faster than normal. Using a heavy weight won't allow you to achieve this, and it can also lead to injury. But even though the weight will be such that you can perform considerably more reps than usual, reps should stay in the range of three to five. In other words, you will not train to failure when doing ballistic reps. Again, the objective is to move the weight very quickly on every rep of every set to increase muscular power; doing too many reps will fatigue the muscles and slow the speed of the reps near the end of the set, defeating the purpose. And because you need to minimize fatigue when training for power, rest periods between sets should be at least two minutes.

As with slow-rep training, you should use ballistic-rep sets only occasionally; normal-speed reps should make up the majority of your sets. When implementing this technique into a workout, select just one or two exercises and do three or four sets of ballistic reps.

VARIABLE-SPEED SETS

As mentioned previously, variety in training is key to ensuring long-term progress, and rep speed is certainly not the exception to this rule. Using only one rep speed in your training will allow your muscles to adapt to the predictable stimulus, which can lead to plateaus in results. You should sprinkle ballistic and slow-rep sets into your program on a continual basis, but a more creative way to spark gains in size and strength is to occasionally do slow-, fast-, and normal-speed reps in a single set. This technique is known as variable-speed sets.

In each variable-speed set, you perform a third of the reps explosively, a third very slowly, and a third at a moderate speed (your normal rep speed). Sets of 15 reps work well with this technique because it breaks down easily to five reps at each speed. As with ballistic reps, machine exercises tend to be safer, though you can use free-weight movements too, so long as you use caution while doing the fast reps (that is, don't let the weight leave your hands at the top of the rep).

Weight selection is key here; the resistance should be neither too light nor too heavy. Thus, select a weight with which you can do 20 to 25 normal-speed reps. Do the first five reps as fast as possible, do the second five slowly (five seconds up, five seconds down), and do the final five reps at normal speed. Because performing sets in this manner will tax the muscles in a different manner than you're probably used to, rest two or three minutes between each set to allow for ample recovery. And again, use variable-speed sets only occasionally by doing three sets of them for only one exercise of each muscle group.

STATIC CONTRACTIONS

This technique involves not moving the weight at all—that is, holding one position statically for an extended time. As with slow reps, a muscle's time under tension can be maximized with static contractions to increase the size of muscles. The redeeming quality of static contractions is that the sticking point (the weakest point of the ROM) is eliminated, which allows you to overload the muscle more than you'd normally be able to do.

To perform a static-contraction set, select a weight that's significantly heavier than you would normally use for the particular exercise, and have a spotter help you lift the weight to a point about two to four inches from the full-contraction point of the movement. For example, on biceps curls and presses (either for chest or shoulders), it will be just short of the top position. On pull-downs, it will be just shy of the bottom position. At that point, hold the weight without assistance for 10 to 20 seconds, then have your spotter help you return the weight to a racked position. Once you can hold a weight for more than 20 seconds, it's time to increase the weight. After two sets of static contractions, do three full-ROM sets of that exercise as well as other full-ROM exercises for that muscle group to ensure a well-rounded workout.

NEGATIVES

The positive portion of the rep is the primary focus of most trainees, though the negative is just as crucial in achieving muscular size and strength. In fact, research shows that the negative portion, more so than the positive, stimulates the production of insulin-like growth factor-1 (IGF-1), a protein hormone with substantial anabolic effects in adults. This is why doing sets that concentrate solely on the negative are beneficial to many people.

Doing negatives requires an attentive, trustworthy spotter, first and foremost, since he or she will actually do most of the positive portion of each rep for you. Choose a weight that's heavier than you'd normally use for a straight set of the chosen exercise (you can use negatives on virtually any exercise). When you train with negative reps, the load should be about 130 percent of your one-repetition maximum (1RM) for the exercise you're training. For each rep, perform the negative on your own, lowering (or raising, depending on the exercise) the weight very slowly. It should take you three to five seconds to complete the negative rep. If you can resist the weight for longer than five seconds, add more weight. If you can't resist the weight for at least three seconds, reduce the weight. Perform three sets of four to six negative reps on such major lifts as bench presses, overhead presses, lat pull-downs, and barbell curls. Follow the negative sets with two sets of regular reps using a weight that's about 75 to 80 percent of your 1RM.

You can also perform negatives unilaterally (one arm or one side at a time), which promotes balance (because a strong arm won't be able to compensate for a weak one) and provides a means of doing negatives without a spotter. Dumbbell exercises are ideal for unilateral negatives. On a dumbbell curl, for example, select a heavy dumbbell and lower it slowly through the negative with your right arm, then use your left arm to lift the right arm and the weight through the positive portion. You can do the same on any number of dumbbell exercises, such as one-arm rows for the back, lateral raises for the shoulders, and one-arm overhead extensions for the triceps.

Machines work well for unilateral negatives too. For example, on Smith machine presses you can lower the bar through the negative using only one arm, then lift through the positive with either the opposite arm or both arms. The same applies for cambered machines for the chest, back, shoulders, or arms. You can even use cable exercises, such as rows for the back or press-downs for the triceps.

Both dumbbell curls and Smith machine presses present a novel approach to negative training, a variation called split-rep training, where for each rep both the negative and positive are accentuated, albeit by opposite arms or sides. Going back to the curl example, one complete split rep would consist of lowering the dumbbell slowly with the right arm, transferring it to the left hand, then curling it up with that arm with a normal-speed rep. This way you execute a negative with one arm and a positive with the other. After completing a set, you would alternate arms, doing the negative with the left and the positive with the right.

As with any advanced technique, use negatives in moderation, not in every workout. Limit your use of them to the first two sets of an exercise, and don't do negatives in every workout. Instead, do them as an occasional tool for sparking increases in muscular strength and growth.

PREEXHAUSTION

This technique isn't so much an exercise technique as it is a flip-flopping of exercise order. Chapter 3 advises you to perform compound exercises before isolation movements when training the chest, back, and shoulders. The preexhaust method is the one exception to this rule. It involves beginning your workout with an isolation exercise (a fly or crossover for the chest, straight-arm pull-down for the back, or lateral raise for the shoulders), then following that up with a compound movement (some form of press for the chest, pull-down or row for the back, or overhead press or upright row for the shoulders).

The logic behind preexhaustion is that on compound exercises for the upper body, the arms tend to tire out before the chest, back, or shoulders do. For example, you might fail at eight reps of seated rows because your biceps were too fatigued to go on, even though your back muscles still had plenty of energy left in them and could have done several more reps. In this case, the effectiveness of the exercise is diminished because the whole point of rowing exercises is to fatigue the latissimus, not the biceps.

However, if you do an exercise that isolates the back muscles from the biceps (such as straight-arm pull-downs or pull-backs) before doing rows, the larger muscles (latissimus) will be prefatigued before the compound exercise and thus more likely to fail at about the same time as the biceps, if not sooner. See table 10.7 for a sample preexhaust workout for the back. This concept applies to doing dumbbell flys or cable crossovers before flat, incline, or decline presses for chest or lateral raises before overhead presses for shoulders. See tables 10.8 and 10.9 for sample preexhaust workouts for the chest and shoulders. You can use preexhaustion occasionally to add variety to your workout or to offset your arms if they are acting as a weak link in compound chest, back, and shoulder exercises.

TABLE 10.7 Sample Back Preexhaust Workout

Exercise	Sets	Reps
Straight-arm pull-down	4	10-12
Wide-grip lat pull-down	4	6-8
T-bar row	4	8-10

TABLE 10.8 Sample Chest Preexhaust Workout

Exercise	Sets	Reps
Cable crossover	4	10-12
Smith machine bench press	4	6-8
Dumbbell incline press	4	8-10

TABLE 10.9 Sample Shoulder Preexhaust Workout

Exercise	Sets	Reps
Cable lateral raise	4	10-12
Smith machine overhead press	4	6-8
Barbell upright row	4	8-10

PYRAMIDING

A standard lifting pyramid is a manner of increasing the amount of weight you use on each successive set while decreasing the number of reps you perform. Theoretically, you shouldn't be able to do as many reps with a heavier weight unless you're terminating sets well before reaching failure. Many advanced lifters and athletes use this technique to ensure progressive overload and to incorporate a variety of rep schemes. In the course of one exercise you might pyramid from 15 to 20 reps down to 6. However, a pyramid can also be more gradual than that, perhaps increasing weight by only 10 to 20 percent so that the rep scheme for a particular exercise might entail, set by set, 12, 10, 8, and 6 reps.

The opposite of a standard pyramid is a reverse pyramid. As the name implies, in each successive set of a given exercise, the weight decreases as the reps increase. Thus, a reverse pyramid might look something like this: 200 pounds for 6 reps in set 1; 180 pounds for 8 reps in set 2; 160 pounds for 10 reps in set 3; 140 pounds for 12 reps in set 4. One of the major benefits of doing a reverse pyramid is that the heaviest sets are performed when your muscles are still fresh and able to handle maximum loads to increase muscular strength and size.

Table 10.10 provides a sample workout with standard and reverse pyramids. As you'll notice, both standard and reverse pyramids are employed for each muscle group (triceps and biceps) in this particular example.

TABLE 10.10 **Arm Pyramid**

For the lying barbell extension and the alternating dumbbell curl, perform a reverse pyramid by decreasing the weight by 10 to 20 percent on each set. For the other exercises, complete a standard pyramid by increasing the weight every set by 10 to 20 percent. Rest 1 to 2 minutes between each set.

Exercise	Reps for set 1	Reps for set 2	Reps for set 3	Reps for set 4
TRICEPS				
Close-grip bench press	12	10	8	6
Lying barbell extension	6	8	10	12
Overhead dumbbell extension*	12	10	8	
BICEPS				
Barbell curl	12	10	8	6
Alternating dumbbell curl	6	8	10	12
Hammer curl*	12	10	8	

*The last exercise for each muscle group includes only 3 sets to keep the total volume in check to avoid overtraining.

Incorporating both types in the same workout will allow you to reap the benefits of each while promoting variety in your training that will lead to better long-term gains in size and strength and minimize training plateaus.

CHEATING REPS

Although strict exercise form is recommended for a majority of your sets, cheating from time to time will allow you to use more weight than normal to spark gains in size and strength. A cheating rep simply involves straying from proper form—putting a little body English into a rep—to help create momentum and get you past a sticking point.

For example, say you normally use 100 pounds for barbell curls for 10 strict reps. You can use 120 to 150 pounds for the same number of reps by thrusting your hips forward at the bottom portion of each rep to move the weight through the sticking point. You would do the top half of the ROM much more strictly because that's where your biceps are strongest; as a result, you've just overloaded your biceps 20 to 50 percent through the strongest portion of their ROM, which can lead to significant increases in size and strength. Another way to implement cheating reps is to do strict reps until failure and then finish the set with several body English reps. That way, you reap the benefits of proper exercise form while extending the set past failure to boost intensity.

Of course, you should use cheating reps only sparingly. And when using them, don't do more than one set of cheating reps per exercise, and make sure that even though you're compromising technique you're not exposing yourself to injury. In fact, some exercises simply don't lend themselves to cheating reps because the risk of injury is too great. You can do exercises such as curls, lateral raises, cable press-downs, and lat pull-downs in a cheating fashion while still minimizing injury risk. However, cheating on barbell presses (flat bench, incline, decline, overhead), bent-over barbell rows, or other heavy compound free-weight exercises is not advised. Maintain strict form on all such exercises, and save the cheating reps for isolation moves in which you use a lighter weight.

CHAPTER 11

Tailor-Made Programs

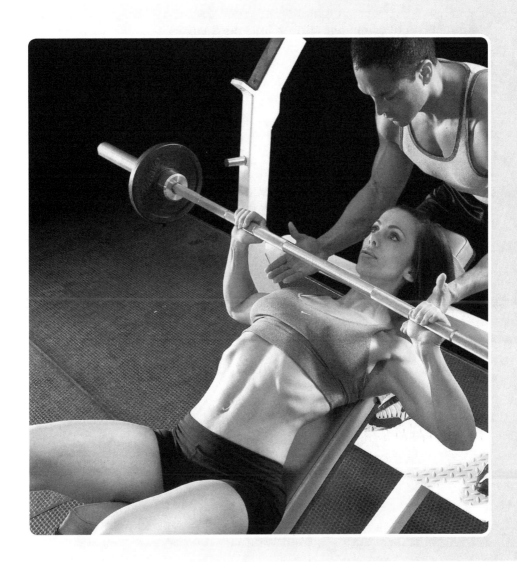

E verything discussed up to this point—muscular anatomy, training concepts, exercise descriptions, and advanced techniques—is a means of building a complete training program. Armed with the information in the first 10 chapters, you should be able to design your own program. But if you'd rather not create your own, we've done the legwork for you.

Because we realize that each person has unique goals, we've drawn up three distinct programs: one that builds maximum size, one that focuses on muscular strength, and one that burns the most calories possible to maximize fat burning. Each program is three months long, consisting of multiple phases that alter the exercises performed, training volume, and intensity to keep your muscles from getting accustomed to one particular stimulus. Over the course of nine months, you can do all three programs if you wish; together they form a longer periodized program in which training objectives change throughout the year.

Within each program, you have options—virtually every exercise can be substituted for another one of your choice. For the most appropriate alternatives, refer to the Substitutes section of each exercise in chapters 4 through 9. In addition to switching out exercises, you can vary the days you train from what the following programs suggest.

MASS-BUILDING PROGRAM

The 12-week mass-building program presented in table 11.1 (beginning on page 202) consists of three four-week phases. As you'll see, the program incorporates a myriad of rep ranges (high reps, low reps, and moderate reps) to subject the muscles to heavy weights, lighter weights, and everything in between. Exposure to a variety of weights will keep the muscles from hitting a plateau, allowing the muscles to continue to grow throughout the program's 12 weeks. Of course, strength and endurance will be enhanced to some extent in this program, but the overriding objective is size.

Phase 1 Weeks 1 to 4 emphasize low reps on basic multijoint exercises (with the exception of biceps), which hit multiple muscle groups to increase strength as well as overall muscle size. The strength gains made during this phase will allow you to lift more weight during the last two phases, which will enhance the muscular growth you'll experience over the long term. Train by using a push–pull split in phase 1, training each muscle group twice a week.

In weeks 1 and 2 of phase 1, reps remain in the range of 6 to 7; perform one drop set on the last set of the first and last exercise for each muscle group to increase intensity. In weeks 3 to 4, reps for the primary lifts of each muscle group drop to the 3 to 5 range, with one added twist—a drop set. After the last heavy set of each primary lift, decrease weight considerably and immediately perform 25 reps of that exercise. Besides increasing muscular endurance, this practice boosts strength and mass, as reported in a recent issue of the *Journal of Strength and Conditioning Research* (Goto et al. Muscular adaptations to combinations of high- and low-intensity resistance exercises. *J Strength Cond Res.* 2004 Nov; 18(4): 730-7). (When researchers had trained lifters perform sets in the 3- to 5-rep range, they made significantly greater gains in strength and muscle mass when they added one set of 25 reps immediately after the last set.) This set of high reps also prepares your muscles for the high-rep training in phase 2.

Phase 2 Reps increase substantially in weeks 5 to 8. The most important thing for making continued gains in muscle mass is change. The body adapts quickly to the same program; thus the reps at this stage change from low to high to shock the muscle into further growth. Phase 2 switches to a two-day split to allow different muscle groups to be trained on different days and with different muscles. You still train each muscle group twice a week, which means you'll still do four workouts per week.

In the first two weeks of phase 2, you include more isolation exercises but still start workouts with compound movements. The first exercise (a compound move) is lower in reps, whereas the isolation moves incorporate high reps. During weeks 7 and 8, implement the preexhaust technique, in which you perform isolation exercises first with low reps followed by compound movements with high reps.

Phase 3 Weeks 9 to 12 call on high-intensity techniques to force the muscles to grow even more. This phase changes rest periods between sets substantially by incorporating tri-sets in the first two weeks and giant sets in the last two weeks. This is important for keeping growth hormone levels high, which both maximizes muscle growth and reduces body fat so that you end the program larger and leaner. Do a four-day split, reducing training frequency to once per week for each muscle group to provide your muscles more time to recover from the aforementioned high-intensity techniques.

In the first two weeks, do tri-sets that start with compound exercises for low reps (6 on the first exercise) and move to isolation exercises for higher reps (12 reps on the second exercise, 25 on the third). This variety of rep ranges enhances muscular strength, mass, and endurance. In the last two weeks of the program, do giant sets in which reps and exercise order are reversed—isolation movements with high reps precede compound moves with low reps.

TABLE 11.1 Mass-Building Program

PHASE 1: WEEKS 1-2				

WORKOUT 1: MONDAY, THURSDAY (PUSH WORKOUT)

Muscle group	Exercise	Sets	Reps	Rest
Chest	Incline barbell press	4	6-7*	2-3 min
	Dumbbell press—flat bench	4	6-7	2-3 min
	Cable crossover	3	6-7*	2-3 min
Shoulders	Dumbbell shoulder press	3	6-7*	2-3 min
	Dumbbell upright row	3	6-7	2-3 min
	Lateral raise	3	6-7*	2-3 min
Trapezius	Dumbbell shrug	3	6-7*	2-3 min
Triceps	Bench press—close-grip	3	6-7*	2-3 min
	Bench dip	3	6-7*	2-3 min

WORKOUT 2: TUESDAY, FRIDAY (PULL WORKOUT)

Muscle group	Exercise	Sets	Reps	Rest
Back	Bent-over barbell row	4	6-7*	2-3 min
	Lat pull-down	4	6-7	2-3 min
	One-arm dumbbell row	4	6-7*	2-3 min
Biceps	Barbell curl	4	6-7*	2-3 min
	Incline dumbbell curl	3	6-7*	2-3 min
Forearms	Barbell wrist curl	3	6-7*	2-3 min

*On the last set, perform one drop set.

PHASE 1: WEEKS 3-4				

WORKOUT 1: MONDAY, THURSDAY (PUSH WORKOUT)

Muscle group	Exercise	Sets	Reps	Rest
Chest	Barbell bench press	4	3-5	2-3 min
		1	25	2-3 min
	Smith machine decline press	4	4-6	2-3 min
	Incline dumbbell press	3	4-6	2-3 min
Shoulders	Barbell overhead press	4	3-5	2-3 min

Muscle group	Exercise	Sets	Reps	Rest
		1	25	2-3 min
	Dumbbell overhead press	3	4-6	2-3 min
	Upright row	3	4-6	2-3 min
Trapezius	Barbell shrug	3	4-6	2-3 min
Triceps	Bench press—close-grip	4	3-5	2-3 min
		1	25	2-3 min
	Dip—narrow grip	3	6-8	2-3 min

WORKOUT 2: TUESDAY, FRIDAY (PULL WORKOUT)

Muscle group	Exercise	Sets	Reps	Rest
Back	Bent-over barbell row	4	3-5	2-3 min
	Reverse-grip pull-down	4	4-6	2-3 min
	Seated cable row	4	4-6	2-3 min
Biceps	Barbell curl	4	3-5	2-3 min
	Hammer curl	3	4-6	2-3 min
Forearms	Standing wrist curl	3	4-6	2-3 min

PHASE 2: WEEKS 5-6

WORKOUT 1: MONDAY, THURSDAY

Muscle group	Exercise	Sets	Reps	Rest
Chest	Incline barbell press	4	8-10	2 min
	Dumbbell fly	4	15-20	2 min
	Cable crossover	4	25-30	2 min
Back	Pull-up—wide-grip	4	to failure	2-3 min
	One-arm dumbbell row	4	15-20	2 min
	Straight-arm pull-down	4	25-30	2 min

WORKOUT 2: TUESDAY, FRIDAY

Muscle group	Exercise	Sets	Reps	Rest
Shoulders	Barbell overhead press	4	8-10	2 min
	Dumbbell lateral raise	3	15-20	2 min
	Bent-over dumbbell lateral raise	3	25-30	2 min

(continued) ▶

TABLE 11.1 PHASE 2: WEEKS 5-6: WORKOUT 2 *(continued)*

Muscle group	Exercise	Sets	Reps	Rest
Trapezius	Smith machine shrug	4	15-20	2 min
Triceps	Bench press—close-grip	3	8-10	2 min
	Lying barbell extension	3	15-20	2 min
	Cable press-down	3	25-30	2 min
Biceps	Barbell curl	3	8-10	2 min
	Barbell preacher curl	3	15-20	2 min
	Concentration curl	3	25-30	2 min
Forearms	Standing wrist curl	2	15-20	1-2 min
	Standing reverse wrist curl	2	25-30	1-2 min

PHASE 2: WEEKS 7-8

WORKOUT 1: MONDAY, THURSDAY

Muscle group	Exercise	Sets	Reps	Rest
Chest	Incline dumbbell fly	4	8-10	2 min
	Incline dumbbell press	3	15-20	2 min
	Barbell bench press	3	25-30	2 min
Back	Straight-arm pull-down	4	8-10	2 min
	Lat pull-down	4	15-20	2 min
	Bent-over barbell row	4	25-30	2 min

WORKOUT 2: TUESDAY, FRIDAY

Muscle group	Exercise	Sets	Reps	Rest
Shoulders	Cable lateral raise	3	8-10	2 min
	Dumbbell overhead press	3	15-20	2 min
	Smith machine overhead press	3	25-30	2 min
Trapezius	Dumbbell shrug	3	25-30	2 min
Triceps	Lying barbell extension	3	8-10	2 min
	Bench dip	3	15-20	2 min
	Bench press—close-grip	3	25-30	2 min
Biceps	Cable concentration curl	3	8-10	2 min
	Incline dumbbell curl	3	15-20	2 min
	Barbell curl	3	25-30	2 min

PHASE 3: WEEKS 9-10

WORKOUT 1: MONDAY

Muscle group	Exercise	Sets	Reps	Rest
Chest	Tri-set	5		2 min between tri-sets
	Incline Smith machine press		6	
	Dumbbell press—flat bench		12	
	Cable crossover		25	

WORKOUT 2: TUESDAY

Muscle group	Exercise	Sets	Reps	Rest
Shoulders	Tri-set	4		2 min between tri-sets
	Dumbbell overhead press		6	
	Dumbbell lateral raise		12	
	Bent-over dumbbell lateral raise		25	
Trapezius	Tri-set	2		2 min between tri-sets
	Smith machine shrug		6	
	Smith machine shrug (behind the back)		12	
	Dumbbell shrug		25	

WORKOUT 3: THURSDAY

Muscle group	Exercise	Sets	Reps	Rest
Back	Tri-set	5		2 min between tri-sets
	Seated cable row		6	
	Lat pull-down		12	
	Straight-arm pull-down		25	

WORKOUT 4: FRIDAY

Muscle group	Exercise	Sets	Reps	Rest
Triceps	Tri-set	3		2 min between tri-sets
	Bench press—close-grip		6	

(continued) ▶

TABLE 11.1 PHASE 3: WEEKS 9-10: WORKOUT 4 *(continued)*

Muscle group	Exercise	Sets	Reps	Rest
Triceps, *cont.*	Seated overhead extension		12	
	Cable press-down (rope)		25	
Biceps	Tri-set	3		2 min between tri-sets
	Barbell curl		6	
	Seated incline curl		12	
	Cable concentration curl		25	
Forearms	Tri-set	2		2 min between tri-sets
	Standing reverse curl		6	
	Standing wrist curl		12	
	Standing reverse wrist curl		25	

PHASE 3: WEEKS 11-12

WORKOUT 1: MONDAY

Muscle group	Exercise	Sets	Reps	Rest
Chest	Giant set	4		2 min between giant sets
	Machine fly		30	
	Cable crossover		20	
	Incline dumbbell press		10	
	Smith machine bench press		5	

WORKOUT 2: TUESDAY

Muscle group	Exercise	Sets	Reps	Rest
Back	Giant set	4		2 min between giant sets
	Straight-arm pull-down		30	
	Seated cable row		20	
	Lat pull-down		10	
	Machine row		5	

WORKOUT 3: THURSDAY				
Muscle group	**Exercise**	**Sets**	**Reps**	**Rest**
Shoulders	Giant set			2 min between giant sets
	Cable lateral raise	3	30	
	Bent-over dumbbell lateral	3	20	
	Smith machine upright row	3	10	
	Smith machine overhead press	3	5	
WORKOUT 4: FRIDAY				
Muscle group	**Exercise**	**Sets**	**Reps**	**Rest**
Triceps	Giant set	3		2 min between giant sets
	Overhead cable extension (rope)		30	
	Cable press-down (rope)		20	
	Lying barbell extension		10	
	Smith machine bench press—close grip		5	
Biceps	Giant set	3		2 min between giant sets
	Concentration curl		30	
	Cable curl		20	
	Barbell preacher curl		10	
	Barbell curl		5	
Forearms	Giant set	2		2 min between giant sets
	Seated wrist curl		30	
	Seated reverse wrist curl		20	
	Standing wrist curl		10	
	Barbell reverse curl		5	

STRENGTH PROGRAM

As in any good strength program, the core component for our strength program is heavy lifting. But the lifting parameters are different than they are for sheer muscle building. When training for strength, you don't want your body to be as fatigued as when hypertrophy is your overriding goal, because getting stronger requires you to lift near-maximal weight during your workouts. You can't do this in an exhausted state. It's important that you not overtrain with excessive volume.

The goal of this program is to gain strength on one major exercise per muscle group: bench press for the chest, bent-over barbell row for the back, barbell overhead press for the shoulders, barbell curl for the biceps, and close-grip bench press for the triceps. These are your core compound exercises—the ones that allow you to lift the most weight—for each major muscle group.

Testing Your Strength   At the start of the program, at the end of week 8, and after the 12th and final week, test your strength by determining your one-rep max strength (1RM) for each core compound exercise as a means of measuring your progress. For the first test, be sure your body is fully rested. Rest for a few days before the test and then rest for a few days after the test before beginning the program. For example, test on a Thursday after not having lifted that week, then rest three days and start the program on the following Monday.

In week 8, your test day simply replaces the fourth workout of the week: Friday's fast-rep training day. Then, when the program ends at the end of week 12, rest Saturday, Sunday, and Monday and perform your final test on Tuesday to ensure the most accurate results.

On testing days, don't attempt a true 1RM; estimate it. This method is still highly accurate, but it's easier and safer than a true 1RM. For each exercise, make your best guess about how much weight you can lift for no more than 10 reps (see table 11.2). Attempt as many reps as possible with that weight, and be sure to reach muscle failure. Record the weight and amount of reps completed, and calculate your 1RM using equations in table 11.3.

Training for Strength   The strength program (table 11.4, beginning on page 210) consists of three 4-week phases for a total of 12 weeks. Perform four workouts per week. For workouts 1 to 3 (Monday, Tuesday, and Thursday) during weeks 1 to 4, perform four sets of 6 to 8 reps for each major exercise per muscle group; for workouts 1 to 3 in weeks 5 to 8, do four sets of 4 or 5 reps; and for workouts 1 to 3 during weeks 9 to 12, perform four sets of 2 or 3 reps with the heaviest weight possible. In all 12 weeks, after those four sets, do one more set of the exercise with 60 percent of your 1RM for as many reps as possible, taking the set to failure.

TABLE 11.2 **Test Day Workout**

After 2 or 3 warm-up sets (using a heavier weight on each set), make your best estimate of a weight you can perform for 8 to 10 reps of each exercise and do one set to failure. Note how many reps you were able to perform. Rest at least 5 minutes between exercises.

Muscle group	Exercise	Weight	Sets	Reps	Rest
Chest	Bench press	8- to 10RM	1	8-10	5 min
Back	Barbell row	8- to 10RM	1	8-10	5 min
Shoulders	Overhead press	8- to 10RM	1	8-10	5 min
Biceps	Barbell curl	8- to 10RM	1	8-10	5 min
Triceps	Bench press—close grip	8- to 10RM	1	8-10	5 min

TABLE 11.3 **1RM Estimates**

To estimate your one-rep maximum weight (1RM) for each of the five core exercises, plug the weight you used for the one set to failure into the formula that corresponds to the number of reps you performed.

Number of reps	Equation for 1RM
6	Weight (pounds) $\times$ 1.21 = 1RM
7	Weight (pounds) $\times$ 1.24 = 1RM
8	Weight (pounds) $\times$ 1.27 = 1RM
9	Weight (pounds) $\times$ 1.30 = 1RM
10	Weight (pounds) $\times$ 1.33 = 1RM
11	Weight (pounds) $\times$ 1.36 = 1RM
12	Weight (pounds) $\times$ 1.39 = 1RM

After the core exercise is an assisting movement to support strength improvements. For the chest, the bench press is the major strength movement; the dumbbell press is the assisting exercise. Use the rest-pause technique (see chapter 10 page 188) on the assisting move, doing three rest-pauses per set. The workout concludes with a finishing movement, a single-joint exercise (with the exception of lat pull-downs for the back) that directly works your target muscle.

During all weeks, except week 8 (which is a test week), do speed-rep training for all muscle groups as your fourth workout (Friday) of the week. Speed work is an important component of building strength. By improving your explosive power, you improve the amount of weight you can push.

TABLE 11.4   Strength Program

WORKOUT 1: MONDAY (CHEST)						
Muscle group	**Exercise**	**Notes**	**Resistance**	**Sets**	**Reps**	**Rest**
Chest	Barbell bench press	(Warm-up)	50% 1RM	1	10	1 min
			60% 1RM	1	6	2 min
			70% 1RM	1	4	2 min
	Barbell bench press	Weeks 1-4	80% 1RM	4	6-8	2-3 min
		Weeks 5-8	85-90% 1RM	4	4-5	2-3 min
		Weeks 9-12	95% 1RM	4	2-3	2-3 min
		Weeks 1-12	60% 1RM	1	To failure	2-3 min
	Dumbbell press (flat bench or incline)[1]		6 RM	2	5-6, 2-3, 2-3, 2-3[2]	2 min
	Dumbbell fly (incline or flat)[1]		8-10 RM	2	8-10	2 min
WORKOUT 2: TUESDAY (SHOULDERS, BACK, TRAPEZIUS)						
Muscle group	**Exercise**	**Notes**	**Resistance**	**Sets**	**Reps**	**Rest**
Shoulders	Barbell overhead press	(Warm-up)	50% 1RM	1	10	1 min
			60% 1RM	1	6	2 min
			70% 1RM	1	4	2 min
	Barbell overhead press	Weeks 1-4	80% 1RM	4	6-8	2-3 min
		Weeks 5-8	85-90% 1RM	4	4-5	2-3 min
		Weeks 9-12	95% 1RM	4	2-3	2-3 min
		Weeks 1-12	60% 1RM	1	To failure	2-3 min
	Dumbbell overhead press		6 RM	2	5-6, 2-3, 2-3, 2-3[2]	2 min
	Dumbbell lateral raise (or dumbbell upright row)[3]		8- to 10RM	2	8–10	2 min
Back	Barbell bent-over row	(Warm-up)	50% 1RM	1	10	1 min
			60% 1RM	1	6	2 min
			70% 1RM	1	4	2 min
	Barbell bent-over row	Weeks 1-4	80% 1RM	4	6-8	2-3 min
		Weeks 5-8	85-90% 1RM	4	4-5	2-3 min
		Weeks 9-12	95% 1RM	4	2-3	2-3 min

Muscle group	Exercise	Notes	Resistance	Sets	Reps	Rest
		Weeks 1-12	60% 1RM	1	To failure	2-3 min
	Seated cable row (or one-arm dumbbell row)[3]		6RM	2	5-6, 2-3, 2-3, 2-3[2]	2 min
	Lat pull-down[4]		8- to 10RM	2	8–10	2 min
Trapezius	Barbell shrug		6- to 8RM	3	6-8	2 min

WORKOUT 3: THURSDAY (TRICEPS, BICEPS, FOREARMS)

Muscle group	Exercise	Notes	Resistance	Sets	Reps	Rest
Triceps	Barbell bench press—close grip	Warm-up set	50% 1RM	1	10	1 min
			60% 1RM	1	6	2 min
			70% 1RM	1	4	2 min
	Barbell bench press—close grip	Weeks 1-4	80% 1RM	4	6-8	2-3 min
		Weeks 5-8	85-90% 1RM	4	4-5	2-3 min
		Weeks 9-12	95% 1RM	4	2-3	2-3 min
		Weeks 1-12	60% 1RM	1	To failure	2-3 min
	Lying barbell extension (or dumbbell overhead extension)[3]		6RM	2	5-6, 2-3, 2-3, 2-3[2]	2 min
	Cable press-down (or reverse-grip cable press-down)[3]		8- to 10RM	2	8-10	2 min
Biceps	Barbell curl	Warm-up set	50% 1RM	1	10	1 min
			60% 1RM	1	6	2 min
			70% 1RM	1	4	2 min
	Barbell curl	Weeks 1-4	80% 1RM	4	6-8	2-3 min
		Weeks 5-8	85-90% 1RM	4	4-5	2-3 min
		Weeks 9-12	95% 1RM	4	2-3	2-3 min
		Weeks 1-12	60% 1RM	1	To failure	2-3
	Alternating dumbbell curl (or incline dumbbell curl)[3]		6RM	2	5-6, 2-3, 2-3, 2-3[2]	2 min
	Hammer curl		8- to 10RM	2	8-10	2 min

(continued) ▶

TABLE 11.4 WORKOUT 3 *(continued)*

Muscle group	Exercise	Notes	Resistance	Sets	Reps	Rest
Forearms	Standing wrist curl		8- to 10RM	2	8-10	2 min
	Standing reverse wrist curl		8- to 10RM	2	8-10	2 min

[1]Use the opposite bench position for these two exercises each workout and alternate the bench position each week.
[2]On each set, after doing 5 or 6 reps, do 3 rest-pause sets of 2 or 3 reps.
[3]Substitute the listed exercise with the exercise in parentheses every other week.
[4]Alternate between wide-grip overhand and underhand grip every other week.

WORKOUT 4: FRIDAY (FAST-REP TRAINING)

Exercise	Phase	Resistance	Sets	Reps	Rest
Barbell bench press	Phase 1 (weeks 1-6)	50% RM	3	5	2 min
	Phase 2 (weeks 7-12)	60% RM	3	5	2 min
Barbell bent-over row	Phase 1 (weeks 1-6)	50% RM	3	5	2 min
	Phase 2 (weeks 7-12)	60% RM	3	5	2 min
Barbell overhead press	Phase 1 (weeks 1-6)	50% RM	3	5	2 min
	Phase 2 (weeks 7-12)	60% RM	5	3	2 min
Barbell curl	Phase 1 (weeks 1-6)	50% RM	3	5	2 min
	Phase 2 (weeks 7-12)	60% RM	3	5	2 min
Barbell bench press—close grip	Phase 1 (weeks 1-6)	50% RM	3	5	2 min
	Phase 2 (weeks 7-12)	60% RM	3	5	2 min

On your speed training days, do not use heavy weight. For each of your core lifts, perform only four sets. Perform the first set, your warm-up set, with an unloaded bar (a 45-pound Olympic bar with no additional weight) for 10 reps. Perform every rep as fast and explosively as possible. For the three working sets, use only 50 to 60 percent of your 1RM on each exercise for five reps and no more, even if your muscles don't feel as fatigued as they normally do with heavier weight and more reps. Remember that developing strength isn't about total muscular fatigue.

GET-LEAN PROGRAM

The get-lean program (table 11.5) consists of two 6-week phases for a total of 12 weeks. This program maximizes calorie burning and fat loss. Follow a two-day split, training each muscle group twice a week, for a total of four weekly workouts. Training each muscle group more frequently (twice weekly rather than once) helps you burn more calories and makes getting leaner much easier. Intensity-boosting techniques such as drop sets and extended sets are included in the program to further increase calorie burning.

In both phases, heavy days start with basic compound movements. These multijoint exercises help you burn more calories in the gym because using heavy weights has been shown to keep metabolism elevated longer after workouts. Training heavy with compound moves also helps you maintain, if not gain, muscle mass. This is significant because the more lean muscle mass you have, the faster your metabolism will be (which is why mass-gaining programs are often similar to get-lean programs).

Light days involve the use of the preexhaust technique, in which you train an isolation exercise before a compound move. This is an intensity technique that helps you build good muscle that will be revealed as body fat is lost. Also on light days, rest no more than 30 seconds between sets—research shows that short rest, along with using higher reps, burns the most calories during the workout itself.

Phase 1   During weeks 1 to 6, train heavy one day, light the next two, then heavy again on the fourth day. During this time, your heavy days consist of reps in the 8 to 10 range, and you'll perform two drop sets on the last two sets of the last exercise for each muscle group. Light days involve reps in the 20 to 25 range.

Phase 2   In weeks 7 to 12, train opposite of phase 1: light one day, heavy the next two, then light on the fourth day. In these final six weeks, your heavy days consist of reps in the 5 to 7 range for most exercises, except your second exercise for each muscle group, which is an extended set. Your light days consist of sets of 12 to 15 reps.

TABLE 11.5 Get-Lean Program

PHASE 1: WEEKS 1-6				

WORKOUT 1: MONDAY

Muscle group	Exercise	Sets	Reps	Rest
Chest	Barbell bench press	3	8	2 min
	Incline dumbbell press	3	8	2 min
	Smith machine decline press	3	10*	2 min
Shoulders	Smith machine overhead press	3	8	2 min
	Dumbbell overhead press	3	8	2 min
	Smith machine upright row	3	10*	2 min
Trapezius	Barbell shrug	3	8*	2 min
Triceps	Close-grip bench press	3	8	2 min
	Lying barbell extension	3	10*	2 min

*On each of the last two sets, perform two drop sets.

WORKOUT 2: TUESDAY

Muscle group	Exercise	Sets	Reps	Rest
Back	Straight-arm pull-down	3	25	30 sec
	Barbell bent-over row	3	20	30 sec
	Lat pull-down—reverse grip*	3	20	30 sec
Biceps	Incline dumbbell curl	3	20	30 sec
	Barbell preacher curl	3	25	30 sec
Forearms	Standing reverse wrist curl	3	25	30 sec

WORKOUT 3: THURSDAY

Muscle group	Exercise	Sets	Reps	Rest
Chest	Dumbbell fly	3	25	30 sec
	Incline bench press	3	20	30 sec
	Cable crossover	3	25	30 sec
Shoulders	Barbell overhead press	3	20	30 sec
	Bent-over lateral raise	3	25	30 sec
Trapezius	Dumbbell shrug	3	20	30 sec
Triceps	Cable press-down	3	20	30 sec
	Bench dip	3	25	30 sec

WORKOUT 4: FRIDAY				
Muscle group	**Exercise**	**Sets**	**Reps**	**Rest**
Back	One-arm dumbbell row	3	8	2 min
	Lat pull-down—reverse grip*	3	10	2 min
Biceps	Barbell curl	3	8	2 min
	Concentration curl*	3	10	2 min
Forearms	Standing wrist curl*	3	10	2 min

*On each of the last two sets, perform two drop sets.

PHASE 2: WEEKS 7-12

WORKOUT 1: MONDAY

Muscle group	**Exercise**	**Sets**	**Reps**	**Rest**
Chest	Cable incline fly	3	15	30 sec
	Smith machine incline press	3	12	30 sec
	Machine fly	3	15	30 sec
Shoulders	Cable lateral raise	3	15	30 sec
	Dumbbell overhead press	3	12	30 sec
	Cable bent-over lateral raise	3	15	30 sec
Trapezius	Smith machine shrug	3	15	30 sec
Triceps	Dumbbell overhead extension	3	12	30 sec
	Cable press-down (rope)	3	15	30 sec

WORKOUT 2: TUESDAY

Muscle group	**Exercise**	**Sets**	**Reps**	**Rest**
Back	Barbell bent-over row	3	5	2 min
	Extended set	3		
	Lat pull-down (behind the neck)		3-4	–
	Wide-grip lat pull-down (to front)		2-4	–
	Lat pull-down—reverse grip		2-4	2-3 min
	Seated cable row	3	7	2 min
Biceps	Barbell curl (EZ-bar)	3	5	2 min

(continued) ▶

TABLE 11.5 **PHASE 2: WEEKS 7-12: WORKOUT 2** *(continued)*

Biceps *(cont.)*	Extended set	3		
	Incline dumbbell curl		3-4	–
	Seated dumbbell curl		2-4	–
	Standing dumbbell curl		2-4	2-3 min
	Barbell preacher curl	2	7	2 min
Forearms	Seated wrist curl (dumbbell)	3	7	2 min

WORKOUT 3: THURSDAY				
Muscle group	**Exercise**	**Sets**	**Reps**	**Rest**
Chest	Barbell bench press	3	5	2 min
	Extended sets	3		
	Incline dumbbell press		3-4	–
	Dumbbell press—flat bench		2-4	–
	Decline dumbbell press		2-4	2-3 min
	Incline dumbbell fly	3	7	2 min
Shoulders	Barbell overhead press	3	5	2 min
	Extended sets	3		
	Dumbbell bent-over lateral raise		3-4	–
	Dumbbell front raise		2-4	–
	Dumbbell lateral raise		2-4	2-3 min
	Smith machine upright row	3	7	2 min
Trapezius	Extended set	3		
	Smith machine behind-the-back shrug		3-4	–
	Smith machine shrug		2-4	2 min
Triceps	Close-grip bench press	3	5	2 min
	Extended sets	3		
	Press-down—reverse grip		3-4	–
	Overhead cable extension		2-4	–
	Cable press-down (overhand)		2-4	2-3 min
	Lying barbell extension	3	7	2 min

WORKOUT 4: FRIDAY				
Muscle group	**Exercise**	**Sets**	**Reps**	**Rest**
Back	Straight-arm pull-down	3	15	30 sec
	Lat pull-down—wide grip	3	12	30 sec
	One-arm dumbbell row	3	15	30 sec
Biceps	Incline dumbbell curl	3	12	30 sec
	Cable curl	3	15	30 sec
Forearms	Standing reverse wrist curl (dumbbell)	3	15	30 sec

CHAPTER 12

Ready-to-Use Workouts

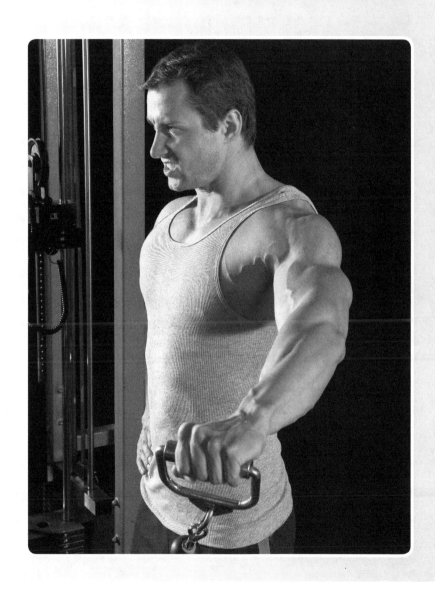

The programs in chapter 11 provide months' worth of workouts to help you meet your fitness goals. But if you're not interested in a major overhaul of your program, this chapter presents individual workouts that you can do occasionally and that fit into virtually any existing program. Exercise selection can vary based on personal preferences (for example, if a workout includes incline barbell press but you'd rather do incline dumbbell press, feel free to switch it out). Alternative movements appear in chapters 4 through 9 under the Substitutes heading for each exercise. Before starting each workout, do at least two warm-up sets of the first exercise.

TROUBLESHOOTING ROUTINES

All lifters have problem areas that they'd like to improve on, whether it be a lack of width or a deficient upper chest. The following routines address the most common trouble spots with exercises that directly target them. Keep in mind that each of these workouts is merely one example of how a particular area can be targeted; by being creative with exercise selection and various set and rep schemes within the general parameters discussed in chapters 1 to 3, you can create endless variations of the following routines.

UPPER CHEST

Explanation
Incline exercises appear early and often to place emphasis on the upper chest.

Rest
Rest 1 to 2 minutes between each set.

Exercise	Sets	Reps
Incline barbell press	4	10, 8, 6, 6*
Superset	3	
Incline dumbbell press		8-10
Incline dumbbell fly		10-12
Cable crossover	3	12-15

*Increase weight every set (pyramid).

LOWER CHEST

Explanation

Decline movements (including dips) take precedence to hit the lower chest.

Rest

Rest 1 to 2 minutes between each set.

Exercise	Sets	Reps
Smith machine decline press	4	8-10
Dumbbell press—flat bench	3	8-10
Weighted dip	3	6-10
Decline cable fly	3	12-15

INNER AND OUTER CHEST

Explanation

Taking a wide grip on the bench press emphasizes the outer chest, while flys and crossovers target both the inner and outer pectorals.

Rest

Rest 1 to 2 minutes between each set.

Exercise	Sets	Reps
Barbell bench press (wide grip)	4	12, 10, 8, 6*
Dumbbell fly	4	8-10
Cable crossover	3	10-12

*Increase weight every set (pyramid).

BACK THICKNESS

Explanation
Rowing exercises are ideal for building a thicker back.

Rest
Rest 1 to 2 minutes between each set.

Exercise	Sets	Reps
Barbell bent-over row	3	6-8
One-arm dumbbell row	3	8-10
Seated cable row	3	10-12
Lat pull-down	3	10-12

BACK WIDTH

Explanation
Pull-ups and pull-downs with a wide grip are the best choices for developing a wider back. Rest-pauses are included on pull-ups to allow more reps to be performed.

Rest
Rest 1 to 2 minutes between each set.

Exercise	Sets	Reps
Pull-up—wide grip	4	To failure*
Lat pull-down (wide grip)	4	8-12
Seated cable row (wide grip)	3	10-12

*On last two sets, perform two rest-pause sets after initially reaching failure.

SHOULDER WIDTH

Explanation

Creating wider shoulders is a matter of building up the middle deltoids via heavy overhead presses (particularly dumbbell or barbell behind-the-neck presses, which allow more middle deltoid involvement), upright rows, and lateral raises. Drop sets on laterals (running the rack) add intensity to the routine.

Rest

Rest 1 to 2 minutes between each set.

Exercise	Sets	Reps
Dumbbell overhead press	4	6-8
Barbell upright row	3	8-10
Dumbbell lateral raise	3	To failure*

*Run the rack on each set.

REAR DELTOIDS

Explanation

Bent-over lateral raises and machine reverse flys place extra focus on the rear deltoids.

Rest

Rest 1 to 2 minutes between each set.

Exercise	Sets	Reps
Barbell overhead press	4	8-10
Dumbbell bent-over lateral raise	4	10-12
Machine reverse fly	3	12-15

FRONT DELTOIDS

Explanation

Arnold presses take the place of regular overhead presses to emphasize the front deltoids; all raises are done to the front, and upright rows emphasize the front deltoids too.

Rest

Rest 1 to 2 minutes between each set.

Exercise	Sets	Reps
Arnold press	4	8-10
Dumbbell upright row	3	8-10
Superset	1	
Cable front raise		10-12
Prone incline barbell front raise		10-12

BICEPS PEAK

Explanation

Concentration curls emphasize the long head, as do hammer curls. When doing dumbbell curls, turn the wrist out at the top and squeeze hard to maximize the contraction.

Rest

Rest 1 to 2 minutes between each set.

Exercise	Sets	Reps
Barbell curl	3	6-8
Incline dumbbell curl	3	8-10
Concentration curl	3	10-12
Cable hammer curl	2	10-12*

*Perform 2 or 3 drop sets at the end of each set.

OUTER TRICEPS

Explanation
All of the following exercises emphasize the triceps lateral head; the close-grip bench press is the major mass builder of the three.

Rest
Rest 1 to 2 minutes between each set.

Exercise	Sets	Reps
Barbell bench press—close grip	4	12, 10, 8, 6*
Lying barbell extension	3	8-10
Cable press-down (rope)	3	10-12**

*Increase weight every set (pyramid).
**Perform 2 or 3 drop sets at the end of last two sets.

UPPER TRICEPS THICKNESS

Explanation
Overhead exercises place a great deal of stress on the triceps long head. Lying extensions with the arms at 45 degrees shift the emphasis there as well.

Rest
Rest 1 to 2 minutes between each set.

Exercise	Sets	Reps
Lying barbell extension*	4	8-10
Overhead dumbbell extension	3	10-12
Overhead cable extension	3	10-12

*Arms at a 45-degree angle to the floor.

FOREARMS

Explanation

In this workout, the lower arms are trained with a variety of wrist positions and through most major forearm motions. Do this routine either on its own or after training biceps.

Rest

Rest 1 to 2 minutes between each set.

Exercise	Sets	Reps
Reverse barbell curl	3	12, 10, 8, 6*
Hammer curl	2	8-10
Seated wrist curl	2	12-15
Standing reverse wrist curl	2	12-15

*Increase weight every set (pyramid).

TRAPEZIUS

Explanation

This routine hits the trapezius from a variety of angles to maximize development. Do the workout either on its own or after training deltoids.

Rest

Rest 1 to 2 minutes between each set.

Exercise	Sets	Reps
Barbell shrug	3	8-10
Dumbbell shrug	3	10-12
Smith machine shrug (behind the back)	3	10-12

BENCH PRESS STRENGTH

Explanation

Enhance bench press strength by keeping reps in the range of 4 to 6. Incline, decline, and fly movements are included in the workout to strengthen all areas of the chest as well as the shoulders, which are heavily involved in benching.

Rest

Rest 2 to 3 minutes between each set.

Exercise	Sets	Reps
Barbell bench press	4	6, 6, 4, 4*
Barbell decline press	4	4-6
Incline dumbbell press	3	6
Dumbbell fly	3	6

*Increase weight every set (pyramid); always use a spotter when doing barbell bench press.

ENDURANCE AND FAT-BURNING ROUTINES

Many people use weightlifting as a way to burn the maximum amount of calories in a workout and thus increase the body's fat-burning potential. That is, often the focus is more on burning calories than on maximizing muscular size and strength. In such workouts, rep ranges needn't be excessively high—sets can range anywhere from 6 to 20 reps and still be effective at burning calories and fat. The more important factor is keeping rest periods brief so that you spend most of the session actually exercising, not resting. Burning maximum calories also requires using compound exercises in which you can lift the most weight and involve the most muscles. The following routines are intense, with a rapid pace that often entails moving from one exercise to the next without resting, either via circuit training or supersets or both.

UPPER-BODY CIRCUIT

Explanation

Because every other set trains a different muscle group, you won't need to rest between sets. Each set alternates from a push to a pull movement to allow each muscle to recover while another is being trained.

Rest

Between sets, rest only as long as it takes to move to the next exercise; rest 1 to 2 minutes between each circuit.

Exercise	Sets	Reps*
Incline dumbbell press	3	15, 12, 10
T-bar row	3	15, 12, 10
Overhead dumbbell press	3	15, 12, 10
Barbell curl	3	15, 12, 10
Lying triceps extension	3	15, 12, 10
Dumbbell shrug	3	15, 12, 10
Standing barbell wrist curl	3	15, 12, 10

Perform one set of each exercise consecutively in each circuit.
*Increase weight each time through the circuit so that you fail at the prescribed number of reps.

MACHINE-ONLY UPPER-BODY CIRCUIT

Explanation

Most weight rooms have areas devoted to selectorized machines, which allow you to move from one exercise to the next in minimal time. Machine exercises can also be a welcome variation if you're accustomed to using only free weights.

Rest

Between sets, rest only as long as it takes to move to the next exercise; rest 1 to 2 minutes between each circuit.

Exercise	Sets	Reps
Machine row	1	10-12
Chest press machine	1	10-12
Machine lateral raise	1	10-12
Machine triceps extension	1	10-12
Machine preacher curl	1	10-12

Perform this circuit 4 or 5 times.

UPPER-BODY SNAKE CIRCUIT

Explanation

In the circuit workouts mentioned previously, the exercise order remains the same each time through the circuit. The result is that one muscle group (whichever goes first) is always trained while it's fresh. A snake circuit reverses the order of exercises each time through so that each muscle receives equal attention. You'll also increase weight on each exercise on successive circuits while *decreasing* rest periods between exercises. This unconventional practice provides a slightly different stimulus each time through as a means of shocking the muscles.

Rest

Rest 1 minute between each exercise during circuit 1, 45 seconds during circuit 2, 30 seconds during circuit 3, and 15 seconds during circuit 4.

Exercise	Reps for circuit 1	Reps for circuit 2*	Reps for circuit 3	Reps for circuit 4*
Dumbbell press	12	10	8	6
Barbell bent-over row	12	10	8	6
Dumbbell lateral raise	12	10	8	6
Alternating dumbbell curl	12	10	8	6
Cable press-down	12	10	8	6

*During circuits 2 and 4, reverse the order of exercises (do cable press-down first and dumbbell press last).

UPPER-BODY SUPERSETS

Explanation

Muscle groups are paired off so that through the course of the workout, you train the chest, back, shoulders, triceps, and biceps in two separate supersets. The chest, back, and shoulders all get paired with one another to promote symmetry and balance.

Rest

Rest 1 to 2 minutes between each superset.

Exercise	Reps for set 1	Reps for set 2	Reps for set 3	Reps for set 4
CHEST AND BACK SUPERSET				
Incline barbell press	12	10	8	6*
Seated cable row	12	10	8	6*
CHEST AND SHOULDER SUPERSET				
Decline barbell press	8-10	8-10	8-10	8-10
Dumbbell overhead press	12	10	8	6*
BACK AND SHOULDERS SUPERSET				
T-bar row	8-10	8-10	8-10	8-10
Upright row	8-10	8-10	8-10	8-10
TRICEPS AND BICEPS SUPERSET 1				
Barbell curl	10	8	6*	
Lying triceps extension	10	8	6*	
TRICEPS AND BICEPS SUPERSET 2				
Dumbbell overhead extension	8-10	8-10	8-10	
Incline dumbbell curl	8-10	8-10	8-10	

*Increase weight every set (pyramid).

CHEST, BACK, AND SHOULDER TRI-SETS

Explanation

Here, the upper body (minus isolation exercises for the arms) is trained thoroughly and intensely via tri-sets in two separate workouts. In the first, each muscle group (chest, back, deltoids) is trained separately with its own series of tri-sets. In the second, each of the three tri-sets includes a chest, back, and shoulder exercise; the order of muscle groups is different in each one.

Rest

Rest 1 to 2 minutes between each tri-set.

EXAMPLE 1		
Exercise	**Sets**	**Reps**
TRI-SET 1: CHEST	3	
Incline barbell press		8
Dumbbell press—flat bench		10-12
Cable crossover		12-15
TRI-SET 2: BACK	3	
Barbell bent-over row		8
Lat pull-down		10-12
Straight-arm pull-down		12-15
TRI-SET 3: SHOULDERS	3	
Smith machine overhead press		8
Dumbbell upright row		10-12
Cable lateral raise		12-15
EXAMPLE 2		
Exercise	**Sets**	**Reps**
TRI-SET 1: CHEST, BACK, SHOULDERS	3	
Incline barbell press		8
Barbell bent-over row		8
Smith machine overhead press		8
TRI-SET 2: BACK, SHOULDERS, CHEST	3	
Lat pull-down		10-12
Dumbbell upright row		10-12
Dumbbell press—flat bench		10-12
TRI-SET 3: SHOULDERS, CHEST, BACK	3	
Cable lateral raise		12-15
Cable crossover		12-15
Straight-arm pull-down		12-15

CHEST AND TRICEPS AND BACK AND BICEPS TRI-SETS

Explanation

In two separate workouts, chest and triceps and back and biceps are trained with typical volume, yet more intensely than when using straight sets. Complete all tri-sets for the chest and back before moving on to the triceps and biceps, respectively.

Rest

Rest 1 to 2 minutes between each tri-set.

CHEST, TRICEPS		
Exercise	**Sets**	**Reps**
CHEST TRI-SET	4	
Smith machine bench press		6-8
Incline dumbbell press		8-10
Cable fly		12-15
TRICEPS TRI-SET	3	
Close-grip bench press		6-8
Dumbbell lying extension		8-10
Dumbbell kickback		12-15
BACK, BICEPS		
Exercise	**Sets**	**Reps**
BACK TRI-SET	4	
Wide-grip pull-up		to failure
Smith machine bent-over row		8-10
Dumbbell straight-arm pull-back		10-12
BICEPS TRI-SET	3	
Barbell curl		6-8
Hammer curl		8-10
Concentration curl		10-12

TIME-SAVING WORKOUTS

You won't always have an hour or more to spend at the gym because of other demands for your time, such as work and family. Fortunately, you can achieve a great workout in 30 minutes or less so long as you manage your time well. The following routines fit a high number of sets into a short time by reducing rest periods and regularly employing supersets. As you'll see, some of them are fairly similar to the endurance (calorie-burning) routines, only with fewer sets to speed things up. When time is of the essence on a particular day, choose one of these workouts instead of skipping the gym.

30-MINUTE UPPER-BODY WORKOUT

Explanation

Do three exercises for each muscle group, but only one set of each. The sequence of exercises (the muscle trained is different each set) is such that minimal rest is required between sets.

Rest

Rest between exercises only as long as it takes you to move from one to the other.

Muscle group	Exercise	Sets	Reps
Chest	Incline barbell press	1	8
Back	Barbell bent-over row	1	8
Shoulders	Dumbbell overhead press	1	8
Triceps	Barbell lying extension	1	8
Biceps	Alternating dumbbell curl	1	8
Chest	Dumbbell press—flat bench	1	10
Back	Lat pull-down	1	10
Shoulders	Cable front raise	1	10
Triceps	Cable overhead extension	1	10
Biceps	Cable curl	1	10
Chest	Dumbbell fly	1	15
Back	Straight-arm pull-down	1	15
Shoulders	Dumbbell lateral raise	1	15
Triceps	Cable press-down—reverse grip	1	15
Biceps	High cable curl	1	15

20-MINUTE CHEST AND BACK WORKOUT

Explanation

Supersetting allows you to train two large body parts with ample volume in a short time.

Rest

Rest 1 minute between each superset.

Exercise	Sets	Reps
Superset	3	
Pull-up—close grip		To failure
Weighted dip		8-10
Superset	3	
Incline dumbbell press		10-12
Seated cable row		10-12
Superset	3	
Lat pull-down		12
Machine press		12

20-MINUTE CHEST, BACK, AND SHOULDER WORKOUT

Explanation

For each exercise, select a weight that will cause you to fail at 10 reps. Do 10 reps, then rest for 30 to 60 seconds. Do as many reps as you can, then rest again. Do this for 5 minutes.

Rest

Rest 1 to 2 minutes between each exercise or muscle group.

Muscle group	Exercise	Time
Chest	Smith machine bench press	5 min
Back	Lat pull-down or seated cable row	5 min
Shoulders	Smith machine overhead press	5 min

20-MINUTE CHEST AND TRICEPS WORKOUT

Explanation

This routine consists of two pairs of chest and triceps exercises. In each pairing, do a set of the chest exercise, then rest and do a set of the triceps exercise, going back and forth until you have performed three sets of each. To save time, do both exercises in each pairing in the same location; in the first pairing, perform both exercises with the same weight (the rep count for chest is considerably higher than for triceps to allow for this).

Rest

Rest 1 minute between each set; the pairs of exercises are *not* to be performed as true supersets.

Exercise pair 1	Sets	Reps
Smith machine bench press	3	15-20
Smith machine bench press—close grip	3	8-10
Exercise pair 2	**Sets**	**Reps**
Incline dumbbell press	3	10-12
Barbell overhead extension*	3	10-12

*Perform on an incline bench.

20-MINUTE BACK AND BICEPS WORKOUT

Explanation

This routine consists of two pairs of back and biceps exercises. In each pairing, do a set of the back exercise, then rest and do a set of the biceps exercise, going back and forth until you have performed three sets of each. To save time, all four exercises in the routine are dumbbell movements, so you can perform them in the same area.

Rest

Rest 1 minute between each set; the pairs of exercises are *not* to be performed as true supersets.

Exercise pair 1	Sets	Reps
Dumbbell bent-over row	3	10-12
Dumbbell curl*	3	10-12
Exercise pair 2	**Sets**	**Reps**
Incline dumbbell row	3	12-15
Incline dumbbell curl*	3	12-15

*Both arms at a time (not alternating).

15-MINUTE ARM WORKOUT

Explanation

Perform the following pairs of exercises as supersets. To save time, each pair of exercises uses the same piece of equipment, which allows you to stay in the same location for both movements.

Rest

Rest 1 minute between supersets.

Exercise	Sets	Reps
SUPERSET 1	2	
Barbell curl		6-8
Lying barbell extension		6-8
SUPERSET 2	2	
Dumbbell overhead extension		8-10
Dumbbell curl*		8-10
SUPERSET 3	2	
Cable curl		12-15
Cable press-down		12-15

*Both arms at a time (not alternating).

ADVANCED WORKOUTS

The one thing that all of the following methods have in common is that they're novel, creative approaches to training. This not only will keep you from getting bored with your workouts, but it will also train your muscles in ways they're not used to; such variety can bring about gains in size, strength, and endurance, depending on the routine. Keep in mind that all of these workouts are of an advanced nature and require a solid training base of at least a year.

HUNDREDS TRAINING

Explanation

Doing sets of 100 reps is a means of both increasing muscular endurance and shocking the muscles to overcome a plateau in strength or size. Train no more than three sets for each muscle group twice a week in this manner (one set each of three different exercises will ensure a well-rounded workout). If you're unaccustomed to high-rep training, do only one exercise (one set of 100 reps) per muscle group initially. Use hundreds training for no more than two weeks at a time in order to avoid overtraining.

For each exercise, select a weight that's approximately 20 to 30 percent of what you would normally use for a set of 10 reps. The goal is to fail initially at around 70 reps—you won't actually be doing 100 reps consecutively. After reaching failure, rest as many seconds as you have remaining reps to reach 100 (for example, if you did 75 reps to failure, rest 25 seconds before starting again). Repeat this until you reach 100 reps, then move on to the next exercise.

In the following workout, the upper body is split into two routines to be performed on separate days to avoid excessive volume in any one workout. Rest at least two days between workouts because the shoulders, biceps, and triceps will need time to recover from the first workout.

Rest

Rest 2 to 3 minutes between exercises or sets.

WORKOUT 1			
CHEST, BACK			
Muscle group	**Exercise**	**Sets**	**Reps**
Chest	Dumbbell press—flat bench	1	100
	Smith machine incline press	1	100
	Fly machine	1	100
Back	Lat pull-down	1	100
	Machine row	1	100
	Straight-arm pull-down	1	100
WORKOUT 2			
SHOULDERS, TRICEPS, BICEPS			
Muscle group	**Exercise**	**Sets**	**Reps**
Shoulders	Smith machine overhead press	1	100
	Dumbbell lateral raise	1	100
Triceps	Dip machine	1	100
	Cable press-down	1	100
Biceps	Barbell curl	1	100
	Machine curl	1	100
Traps	Dumbbell shrug	1	100
Forearms	Standing barbell wrist curl	1	100

70S TRAINING

Explanation

This style of training, like hundreds training, is a way of increasing muscular endurance and providing a shock to the body to elicit gains in size and strength. The only major difference between the two is that you use a significantly heavier weight with 70s—select a resistance that causes you to fail at around 20 reps.

Choose one or two exercises per muscle group. For each set, rep out to failure (again, this should be somewhere around 20 reps), then take a short break (less than a minute) and rep to failure again. Do this until you've reached 70 reps for that exercise. You can use this training method either sporadically when you want to provide a different stimulus to one or more muscle groups or regularly (once or twice per week) for every muscle group for up to four weeks. If you choose the latter, you'll find that the number of sets it takes you to reach 70 reps (assuming you're using the same weight each time) will decrease over time because your muscles will have gained endurance.

Rest

Rest 2 minutes between 70-rep sets.

WORKOUT 1			
BACK, SHOULDERS			
Muscle group	**Exercise**	**Sets**	**Reps**
Back	T-bar row	1	70
	Lat pull-down	1	70
Shoulders	Machine overhead press	1	70
	Dumbbell lateral raise	1	70
WORKOUT 2			
CHEST, TRICEPS, BICEPS			
Muscle group	**Exercise**	**Sets**	**Reps**
Chest	Dumbbell incline press	1	70
	Machine press	1	70
Triceps	Cable press-down	1	70
Biceps	Dumbbell curl*	1	70
Forearms	Barbell reverse curl	1	70

*Both arms at a time (not alternating).

VOLUME TRAINING

Explanation

Even more than hundreds and 70s training, this method further simplifies your workouts. For each workout, perform only one exercise per muscle group. Yet you'll train each exercise with more volume than you've likely ever used for a single movement—up to 15 sets per exercise. The purpose of volume training is to thoroughly exhaust the particular muscle fibers involved in the chosen exercise to increase muscular size.

Train each muscle group twice a week for four weeks with only two exercises (perform one on day 1 of each week, the other on day 2). Each muscle group will need two or three days of rest between workouts. For example, on Monday and Thursday you can train your chest and arms, and on Tuesday and Friday you can train your back and shoulders. The number of sets and reps you perform for each exercise increases every week, from 8 sets of 8 reps in week 1 to 15 sets of 15 reps in week 4. Because the volume at the end of the month is so high, scale down your training (that is, cut your volume in half at the least) over the following couple weeks to allow your body to recover.

Rest

Rest 2 minutes between each set.

	Week 1	Week 2	Week 3	Week 4
MONDAY: CHEST, TRICEPS				
Exercise	**Sets/reps**	**Sets/reps**	**Sets/reps**	**Sets/reps**
Dumbbell press—flat bench	8/8	10/10	12/12	15/15
Cable press-down	8/8	10/10	12/12	15/15
TUESDAY: BACK, SHOULDERS, BICEPS				
Barbell bent-over row	8/8	10/10	12/12	15/15
Dumbbell lateral raise	8/8	10/10	12/12	15/15
Preacher curl	8/8	10/10	12/12	15/15
THURSDAY: CHEST, TRICEPS				
Dumbbell incline fly	8/8	10/10	12/12	15/15
Barbell bench press—close grip	8/8	10/10	12/12	15/15
FRIDAY: BACK, SHOULDERS, BICEPS				
Lat pull-down	8/8	10/10	12/12	15/15
Smith machine overhead press	8/8	10/10	12/12	15/15
Barbell curl	8/8	10/10	12/12	15/15

FOUR-REP TRAINING

Explanation

Training in four-rep increments is a creative means of training for muscular strength, size, and endurance in the same workout. It involves performing sets of 4, 8, 12, and 16 reps for each muscle group so that each area of the body is exposed to heavy-, moderate-, and lightweight training.

You can use four-rep training in one of two ways: Either do four exercises per muscle group (the first one has 4-rep sets, the second 8-rep sets, the third 12-rep sets, and the fourth 16-rep sets) or do two or three exercises per muscle group (four sets each of 4, 8, 12, and 16 reps). The following are examples of both methods for each upper-body muscle group, split into different days.

Rest

Rest 1 to 2 minutes between all sets.

EXAMPLE 1			
CHEST, SHOULDERS			
Muscle group	**Exercise**	**Sets**	**Reps**
Chest	Incline barbell press	3	4
	Dumbbell press—flat bench	3	8
	Decline dumbbell fly	3	12
	Cable crossover	3	16
Shoulders	Barbell overhead press	3	4
	Machine overhead press	3	8
	Dumbbell lateral raise	3	12
	Cable bent-over lateral raise	3	16
BACK, BICEPS, TRICEPS			
Muscle group	**Exercise**	**Sets**	**Reps**
Back	Weighted pull-up	3	4
	Seated cable row	3	8
	Dumbbell straight-arm pull-back	3	12
	Back extension	3	16
Biceps	Barbell curl	2	4
	Dumbbell preacher curl	2	8
	Drag curl	2	12
	Lying cable concentration curl	2	16

(continued)

EXAMPLE 1, *CONTINUED*			
Muscle group	**Exercise**	**Sets**	**Reps**
Triceps	Barbell bench press—close grip	2	4
	Barbell lying triceps extension	2	8
	Cable press-down—reverse grip	2	12
	Cable kickback	2	16

EXAMPLE 2			
CHEST, SHOULDERS			
Muscle group	**Exercise**	**Sets**	**Reps**
Chest	Smith machine incline press	4	4, 8, 12, 16
	Decline dumbbell press	4	4, 8, 12, 16
	Dumbbell fly	4	4, 8, 12, 16
Shoulders	Smith machine overhead press	4	4, 8, 12, 16
	Barbell upright row	4	4, 8, 12, 16
	Cable lateral raise	4	4, 8, 12, 16
BACK, BICEPS, TRICEPS			
Muscle group	**Exercise**	**Sets**	**Reps**
Back	Barbell bent-over row	4	4, 8, 12, 16
	Lat pull-down	4	4, 8, 12, 16
	Straight-arm pull-down	4	4, 8, 12, 16
Biceps	Barbell curl (EZ-bar)	4	4, 8, 12, 16
	Cable preacher curl	4	4, 8, 12, 16
Triceps	Dumbbell lying extension	4	4, 8, 12, 16
	Cable overhead extension	4	4, 8, 12, 16

Appendix: Metric Equivalents for Dumbbells and Weight Plates

The tables here provide conversions for common dumbbell and weight plate increments. For weights not listed here, you can calculate conversions using this equivalent: 1 kilogram = 2.2 pounds.

POUND INCREMENTS CONVERTED TO KILOGRAMS

Pounds	Kilograms
DUMBBELLS	
5	2.3
10	4.5
15	6.8
20	9
25	11.4
30	13.6
35	15.9
40	18.2
45	20.5
50	22.7
WEIGHT PLATES	
2.5	1.1
5	2.3
10	4.5
25	11.4
35	15.9
45	20.5

KILOGRAM INCREMENTS CONVERTED TO POUNDS

Kilograms	Pounds
DUMBBELLS	
2.5	5.5
5	11
7.5	16.5
10	22
12.5	27.5
15	33
17.5	38.5
20	44
22.5	49.5
25	55
30	66
WEIGHT PLATES	
1.25	2.75
2.5	5.5
5	11
10	22
15	33
20	44
25	55

About the Authors

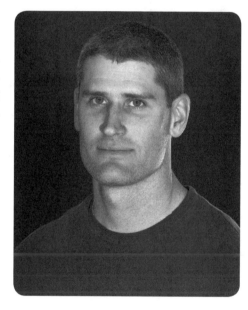

Joe Wuebben serves as senior features editor at *Muscle & Fitness,* the world's largest bodybuilding publication. Having previously worked at *Muscle & Fitness* as a freelance writer and then features editor, he was promoted to his present position in 2007. He has written more than 100 articles dealing with body-part-specific workouts, periodized programs, and advanced training techniques, and he has published in *Muscle & Fitness Hers, Men's Fitness,* and other top publications. Wuebben has twice been cited in the *Best American Sports Writing* anthology (2006 and 2007) for articles in *Muscle & Fitness.*

Wuebben authored *Book of Champions: 40 Years of Mr. Olympia Training Secrets,* which featured workouts and training advice from the all-time great bodybuilders. He earned a bachelor's degree in kinesiology with an emphasis in exercise physiology from Western State College in Gunnison, Colorado. Wuebben lives in Charlotte, North Carolina.

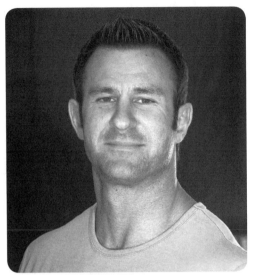

Coauthor **Jim Stoppani, PhD,** is senior science editor at *Muscle & Fitness, Muscle & Fitness Hers,* and *Flex* magazines. One of the foremost researchers in the field of exercise science, Stoppani received his doctorate in exercise physiology from the University of Connecticut. After graduation, he served as a postdoctoral research fellow in the prestigious John B. Pierce Laboratory and department of cellular and molecular physiology at Yale University School of Medicine, where he investigated the effects of exercise and diet on gene regulation in skeletal muscle.

Stoppani was awarded the Gatorade Beginning Investigator in Exercise Science Award in 2002. In 2006, he authored *Encyclopedia of Muscle & Strength* published by Human Kinetics. He is also coauthor of the chapter "Nutritional Needs of Strength/Power Athletes" in the textbook *Essentials of Sports Nutrition and Supplements* (Humana Press, 2008) and is a contributor to the book *Mario Lopez's Knockout Fitness* (Rodale, 2008). He is the personal health and nutrition consultant for numerous celebrity clients, including Dr. Dre and Mario Lopez. Stoppani resides in Los Angeles.

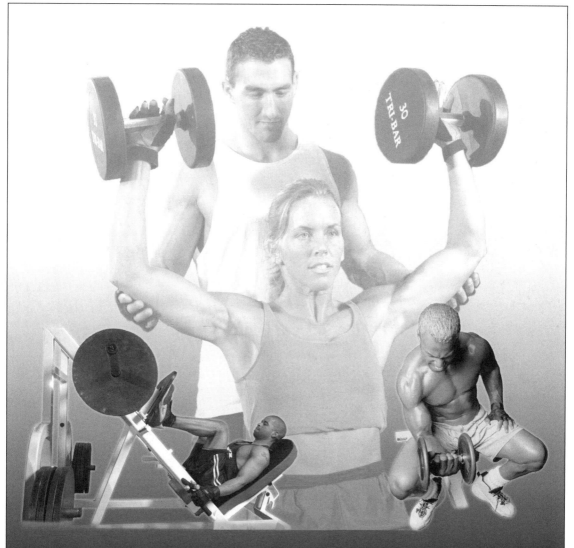